THE COMPLETE BOOK OF
ENERGY MEDICINES

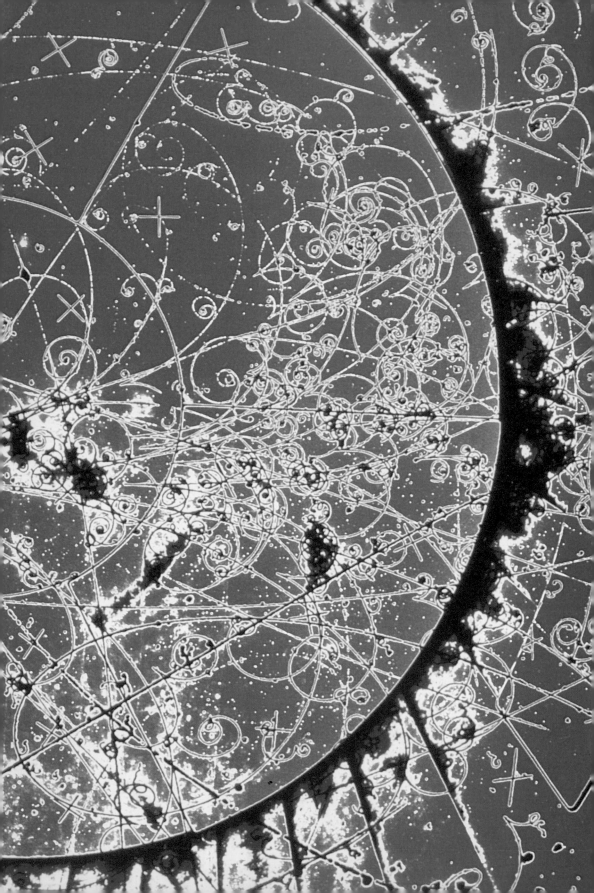

THE COMPLETE BOOK OF

ENERGY MEDICINES

CHOOSING

YOUR

PATH TO

HEALTH

HELEN E. DZIEMIDKO, M.D.

Healing Arts Press
Rochester, Vermont

Healing Arts Press
One Park Street
Rochester, Vermont 05767
www.InnerTraditions.com

Healing Arts Press is a division of Inner Traditions International
Copyright © 1999 by Inner Traditions International
Copyright © 1999 Gaia Books Ltd, London
Text copyright © 1999 by Helen E. Dziemidko

Note to the reader: This book is intended as an informational guide. The therapies, approaches, and techniques described herein are meant to supplement, and not to be a substitute for, professional medical care or treatment. They should not be used to treat a serious ailment without prior consultation with a qualified health care professional.

Library of Congress Cataloging-in-Publication Data

Dziemidko, Helen E.
    The complete book of energy medicines : choosing your path to health / Helen E. Dziemidko ; foreword by Stephan Rechtschaffen.
      p.   cm.
    Includes bibliographical references and index.
    ISBN 0-89281-845-X (alk. paper)
    1. Mental healing. 2. Vital force —Therapeutic use. 3. Alternative medicine. I. Title.
RZ401.D98   1999
615.5—DC21   99-28518
                                      CIP

Printed and bound in Italy

10 9 8 7 6 5 4 3 2 1

Text design and layout by Lucy Guenot
This book was typeset in Sabon and Grotesque

Dedication

✦

To the two souls – who I never met –
whose deaths gave me renewed life.

How to use this book

The aim of this book is to help you to find a complementary therapy that
will help you to heal yourself.

To set the scene, **Part One, Discovering energy,** guides you through theories
about the nature of healing (*What is healing?*), from both orthodox and
alternative perspectives, through the different theories of energy (*The physics
of energy*), both historical and contemporary, and Western and Eastern traditions
(*Traditional views of energy*), to the various ways in which energy is
experienced (*Perceiving energy*).

Part Two, Complementary therapies, helps you to discover the 45 best-known
complementary therapies, giving a brief explanation of origins, how the therapy
works in theory and practice in terms of the subtle body system, what you can
expect if you attend a session, and for what types of ailments the therapy might
be most effective.

Part Three, Flow charts for common ailments, explores, using a simple "Yes"
and "No" format, the most common conditions and gives careful guidance on
what therapy, or therapies, might be best for you, considering the energetic
disturbances at the root of the problem.

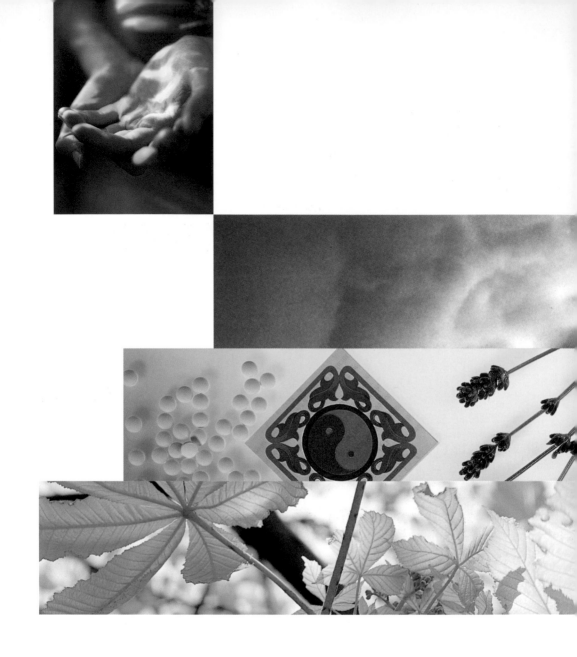

Contents

Part 1
Discovering energy   12

Part 2
Complementary therapies   60

Part 3
Flow charts for common ailments   118

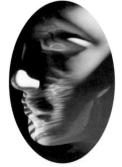

FOREWORD

We each recognize the relationship of energy to our sense of well-being, yet it remains so difficult to define. When we feel good, full of vigor, we feel "energetic", yet when fatigued or ill, we feel low in energy. Each of us seeks more energy, as though we are trying to power our body like an automobile.

In my years at medical school I never heard reference to the body's energy fields. Discussions about energy were left behind in earlier studies of physics. Yet as I progressed it became obvious that people, with almost any illness, seemed depleted, their systems simply seemed to have less energy. As I examined patients in early illness it was obvious that different physiological systems were out of balance, and with further deterioration this imbalance became more widespread. Whether immune, endocrine, neurological, or cardiovascular system, these imbalances would show either over- or under-functioning, indicating too much or too little energy production. To bring these systems into equilibrium required adjusting energy levels into balance.

Yet despite noting what seems obvious about the body's energy, within Western conventional medicine there is no recognition of it, especially the subtle energy systems. As many physicians and healers have begun to recognize, the great need for an inte-grated approach to medicine, including conventional and traditional modalities, understanding the role of the energy fields in healing is essential in developing this "new medicine". So what do we understand about the energy fields and how do we determine their role in physiology and health? As a physician working with an holistic approach to medicine, I've long believed this issue fundamental.

In the space–time continuum we have defined three dimensions of space and one of time. Within the confines of the spatial dimensions we can find the material that makes up the stuff of our bodies. We call this "matter". When this is infused with energy we experience birth of life. Time is the rhythmic dimension of life wherein resides the ebb and flow of energy. Within this temporal realm we find the energetic frequencies that create these energy fields. To understand energy we must delve into the myriad rhythms interwoven on all levels of existence. Modern medicine, in its rush to cure disease, has focused almost exclusively on the body's gross material nature, without attention to temporal rhythms and subtle energy fields, so long part of traditional approaches. We now enter an era where a new medicine emerges to span these disparate approaches. Energy medicine is essential in this.

In this thorough approach to understanding the many forms of the body's energetic fields, Helen Dziemidko explores how self-healing and health interconnect. She has examined the many systems of healing to understand the role of these energy fields in the different functions of the body and how to interact with these to restore balance. Each modality of healing operates on a particular frequency. Matching the appropriate healing approach with any underlying condition is greatly facilitated by her work on energy fields. Dr Dziemidko allows the reader to see this relationship of energy fields in many different conditions, as well as how they operate through different healing approaches.

Stephan Rechtschaffen

Stephan Rechtschaffen, MD, is president and co-founder of the Omega Institute for Holistic Studies in Rhinebeck, NY, the oldest and largest holistic education center, recognized worldwide for its broad-based curriculum in health, psychology, professional trainings, multicultural arts, and spirituality.

INTRODUCTION

During my first few days at medical school, I realized that medicine was not practised in the way that I had imagined. Patients had to be labelled with a recognized disease before they were considered for treatment. This involved tests that were often traumatic and treatments that often were worse, or only marginally better than, the natural course of the illness. If no disease was found the patient was told that nothing was wrong, in spite of their experience to the contrary. The treatments used, mainly drugs and surgery, were often inadequate to control the disease, or produced unacceptable side effects. I found this completely disheartening and nearly gave up my study.

At the same time I was fortunate to discover homeopathy and reflexology. These subtle methods of healing appealed to my imagination as better ways of treating illness. I intensified my interest in alternative medicine after qualifying as a doctor and got the opportunity to train with Dr Julian Kenyon in the newly emerging practice of clinical ecology (the diagnosis and treatment of allergies to food or chemicals). Subsequently, I built up my own practice in Liverpool.

I found the tools of clinical ecology useful but limited in effectiveness, so I developed further skills in nutritional medicine and psychotherapy and trained as a homeopath. Combining these methods did seem to cure people in a more complete way, although a frustratingly large number still did not do well. I was intrigued as to why this should be. This problem affected me personally as well as in my work, as I had my own health difficulties. In 1980 I developed a rare kidney disease that left me with kidney failure and subsequently I had a kidney transplant. This experience gave me my own healing process to explore and in 1990 I stopped practising to do this. I spent three summers at the Omega Institute in New York, where I was able to meet and work with many inspirational teachers in the personal growth movement. These and other experiences elsewhere opened up my approach and understanding of healing. When I returned to work I went into general practice in the National Health Service in the UK. In 1995 a second episode of kidney failure, followed by another transplant, took me deeper into my own experiences of healing, particularly its multidimensional nature.

This book, although ostensibly factual and impersonal, is a reflection of the past twenty years of my life experiences as a doctor, a patient, and as a multidimensional human being.

Dr Helen E. Dziemidko

Part 1
Discovering energy

Drawing on ancient mystical traditions, and scientific knowledge, **Part One** tackles the challenging concepts of what healing is, what energy is, and how the energy that is life is experienced in the body. It describes the nature of the subtle energy field that seems to envelop our physical body. We can then begin to understand how we can activate our own healing through interacting with this energy field. It also discusses the differences in the approach to healing between orthodox and alternative treatment methods, as well as looking at what they have in common and how they can work together. This enables you to make informed and constructive choices when it comes to finding your own path to self-healing.

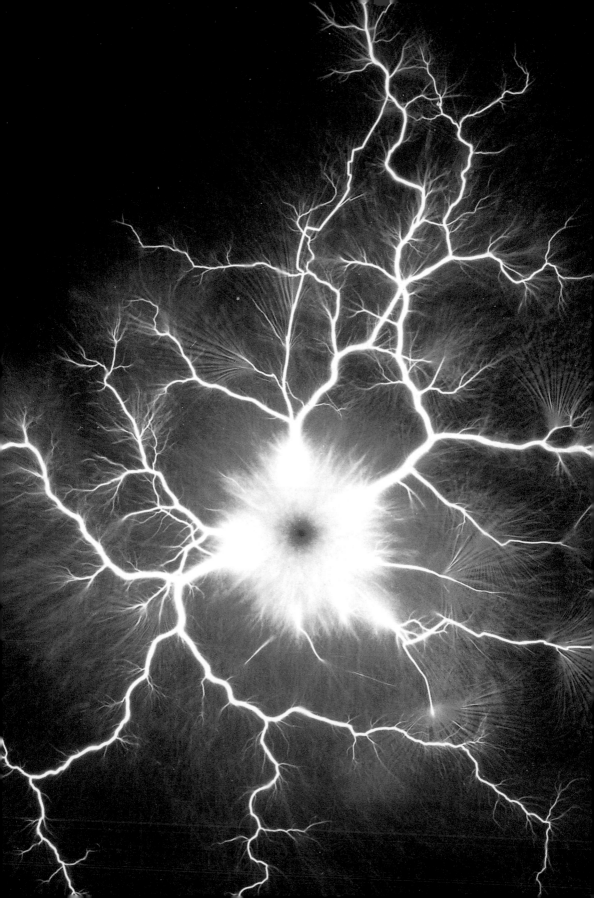

WHAT IS HEALING?

In order to consider what we mean by "healing", in terms of both orthodox and energy medicine, we first need an understanding of how energy healers view the human body and illness.

In everyday language we talk of "having no energy" to describe feelings of unwellness, emotional flatness, or lassitude. It is a common complaint. In fact medical research has shown that one-third of patients attending a doctor's surgery complain of "low energy". But as this complaint is so common, so non-specific, and so ill-understood by orthodox medicine it is dismissed as irrelevant. In contrast, energy medicine bases its treatments on the concept that illness is the primary manifestation of the disturbed energy state.

The dictionary defines energy as a "power", a "force", or "vitality" and these are the meanings that energy has in energy medicine and healing. However energy healing takes the definition further by considering energy in the body as being that which animates the physical body. The word "energy" is used to describe the mystery of life. In other cultures this life energy, or "life force", is well recognized in philosophy and healing traditions. The Chinese have three words to describe different aspects of this energy: "chi", "jing", and "shen"; the Indians call it "prana", the same as their word for breath, or spirit. The use of these words is millennia old. It is only recently, during the last few hundred years, that the concept of body energy in our culture has become eroded in the name of scientific progress.

This life energy generates a field which permeates the physical body and also extends beyond it. Sometimes seen by mystics as a coloured aura, this energy field is traditionally regarded as being made up of separate components – the subtle energy bodies – which relate to different aspects of our being. All these concepts are discussed in more detail on pages 36–40.

It is only recently, during the last few hundred years, that the concept of body energy in our culture has become eroded in the name of scientific progress.

HOW HEALING OCCURS

Everyday healing is a mixture of treatments, both orthodox or complementary, and the workings of the body's own healing abilities. For most illnesses this is satisfactory, but in life-threatening and chronic illnesses, by definition, this is not enough.

The medical science view is that the efficacy of its treatments combined with the body's innate self-regulation processes produces cures. The philosophy of most complementary approaches is to enhance the body's innate ability to heal itself. There is some overlap between these two approaches. For example, body-orientated methods (e.g. osteopathy) are primarily physical, as is orthodox medicine.

Energy healing sees the whole process of healing, whatever the method, as working with the body's energy fields. It may include treatments that work alongside the body's healing process (drugs, surgery, herbs, and supplements) and those that enhance the body's healing process (such as homeopathy). Both ultimately affect the energy bodies.

OUR EXPECTATIONS OF HEALING

For most of us healing means restoration of full physical or psychological health, and this is the aim of orthodox doctors. Energy-based healing aims to restore completion, wholeness, contentment, and joy. Healing may not come in the form we had imagined and may not correspond with a return to good health. Sufferers from chronic, or even terminal, disease sometimes find that healing does not come because they are physically cured but because they see life in a new way, transcending suffering.

Holistic healing

Energy healing differs from orthodox medicine's approach to healing, yet both can contribute to treatment. To deny either approach fails to support "holistic" healing. Each method has advantages and disadvantages; the skill of the holistic approach is knowing how to choose or blend these approaches to the greatest benefit.

On close inspection both the orthodox and energy healing approaches contain the same elements. Orthodox medicine, which attempts to work out what is wrong and "fix it", also relies on trust and respect between doctor and patient, knowing when to allow the body to right itself and allowing its healing mechanisms to complete work started by surgery. Energy healing, which aims to boost the body's self-restorative capacities and not to pre-judge what needs putting right, often uses "fix-it" techniques, such as homeopathy.

All orthodox doctors know of exceptional patients whose healing response is beyond what might reasonably be expected, so they gain a respect for the unknown factor that comes into healing. Each doctor explains this in his or her own way, as it is not something that is taught in medical schools. Energy healing sees these responses as being due to the non-material, or energetic, component of the healing process and aims to maximize this effect.

The orthodox medical approach

Orthodox medicine aims to supply treatment that supports the body while it goes through its self-regulatory repair process. It does not regard the body's natural healing mechanism as an "energy process", but rather as a material-based and scientifically analyzable process.

For acute illnesses there are many examples of how orthodox medicine supports the body's own healing mechanism, to aid restoration of health (see right). Unfortunately recovery from a chronic illness may not be so easy. Such illnesses may persistently undermine health, for example eczema or rheumatoid arthritis, or else may be seriously life-threatening, such as cancer. Modern medicine has a vast array of drugs to "treat" these illnesses. These may remove symptoms and restore apparent physical or psychological wellbeing, but there may also be side effects. Drugs have no effect on the actual elimination of the illness (though this may happen because the body heals itself) and sometimes the side

The body heals itself

Taking out an inflamed appendix removes a potentially lethal source of infection that could cause peritonitis, septicaemia, and even death. The body then heals up the wound of the operation. Antibiotics kill or incapacitate bacteria, so that the body no longer has to defend itself against their invasion. It can then get on with repairing the damage they caused.

effects of a drug may be worse than the disease itself. Also the partial relief of symptoms that drugs bring about may leave other aspects of the disease process unchecked.

Modern orthodox medicine is based on Newtonian physics, with its concept of the universe as a giant clockwork mechanism created by "God". With this view of the world, surgery is simply biological carpentry and plumbing. Drugs seem more sophisticated, but in essence they are biological versions of a lock and key mechanism (see left). In theory this seems a good idea, but the practice of using drugs in healing is fraught with problems such as toxicity and side effects. Also such approaches are rarely curative because the lock and key is almost the last step in the development of illness. Correcting it at this point has no effect on whatever initiated the disease. Ultimately the search for a cure has to leave this simplistic mechanical model. Energy medicine is an attempt to find a more fundamental cure for illness.

The lock and key theory

The concept behind the development of all drugs is to find a chemical shape (the key) that fits into a corresponding template (the lock) on the cell wall accurately. When these two mesh this activates or inactivates one of the processes of the cell, specifically the one that the drug is designed to alter. Morphine is an excellent painkiller and its molecular shape mimics naturally produced painkillers, endorphins. When it enters the body it "fits the lock" that endorphins naturally fill and so triggers the same pain-killing effect as natural chemicals.

TYPES OF ENERGY HEALING

All healing interactions, including orthodox medicine, have three possible components. The first is a physical technique, or medicament, interacting with the physical body to encourage natural healing. For example, a splint supports a broken bone while it heals in the correct position. Acupuncture around the break frees energies and disperses pain. Liver herbs promote the activities of the liver cells and speed up elimination of toxins. These methods have a strong physical effect, though they also work at the levels of the subtle bodies. Anyone can learn and successfully practise these kinds of techniques.

The second component is "magnetic" healing. This is the ability to heal using your own body energy to affect the subtle bodies of a patient. Some people use this gift without a supporting therapeutic method. They are "natural" healers and the method requires no more than the desire to relieve suffering. Others use such healing either consciously or subconsciously while they practise more physical methods. However this type of healing tends to drain energy from the giver to the receiver. Many healers, complementary health practitioners, and orthodox doctors suffer from "burn out" caused in this way.

To avoid draining their own energy, healers need to access "radiant" healing. This third method trains the practitioner to act as an access point for the patient to the limitless supply of energy healing available in the Universe. Energy passes through the practitioner to wherever the patient requires it and can access and heal any part of the subtle bodies as well as the physical body. This is the healing taught to most hands-off and light-touch practitioners. People with natural magnetic healing gifts and those who use magnetic healing should develop radiant healing skills so that healing comes from beyond themselves. Thus they are not only more powerful but can also heal and energize themselves, too. Healers skilled in radiant healing no longer need to use the techniques of their original energy therapy, though they still may use it for maintaining focus and interacting with the patient.

Radiant healing is an opening up to love; a surrendering of the self to the love that fills the Universe, beyond personal experience. This healing is combined with empathy and love, without reservation, for the receiver. It is then combined with intent to direct healing to that person. This is a complete giving of attention to that person, but without investment in the outcome.

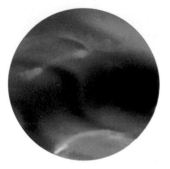

Radiant healing is an opening up to love; a surrendering of the self to the love that fills the Universe, beyond personal experience.

The healer's experience
Both magnetic and radiant healing can produce sensations of warmth, tingling, or expansion in the healer. Others report feelings of coldness or hollowness, while some healers feel or see colours. Very strong movements of energy may make the healer feel faint or as though they were being pushed.

The interpretation of these sensations is individual to each healer and not important. Healing energy

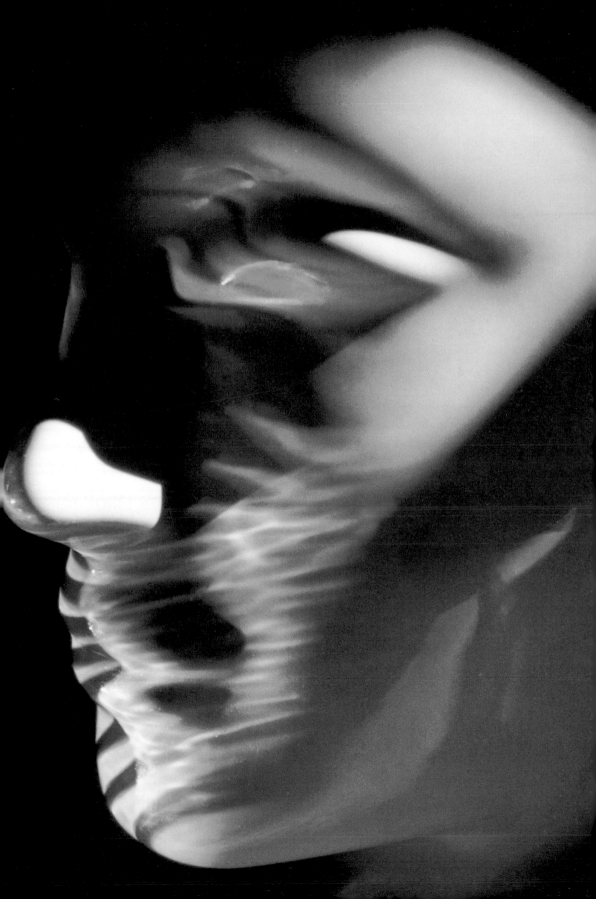

flows to wherever it is needed, to fulfil the body's subconscious needs. Sometimes images or emotions may come to the healer, often expressing lost memories, and sharing this information with the patient may be of value. Healers may also identify their patient's symptoms, or intuitively know what is wrong. This is particularly likely to happen if healing is magnetic. For a radiant healer this would be of no real interest.

The patient's experience

Healing at a deep level may occur during any therapy. First indicators are signs of relaxation (see right). It is not necessary to have faith in a healing technique for it to work; if your healer has faith, this is enough. However an ability to surrender to the illness, the healing process, and the outcome will be most likely to produce healing. Such an attitude may transform your situation into one that gives you inspiration, joy, and a deep experience of love.

THE SCIENCE OF HEALING

Although science does not accept the concepts of healing at an energy level, a great deal of research has been done on well-respected healers and their patients. Much of this work has been done by looking at changes in the electro-encephalogram (EEG), which records the pattern of electrical signals produced in different parts of the brain. These patterns form "brain waves", falling into different categories, depending on wavelength. The EEG can record activities on both sides of the brain. Frequencies of brain waves and the patterns produced on the right side compared with the left side provide information about brain activity.

Brain activity in healing

Powerful healers can generate intense brain-wave patterns, of alpha, theta, and delta waves corresponding to brain states that are most conducive to healing. They can do this at will and in their own personal way, combining elements of being deeply

Signs of relaxation

- *Your breathing pattern will change and deepen – you may sigh or yawn.*

- *You may notice gurgling in your abdomen as the gut relaxes.*

- *You may become cold or flooded with warmth.*

- *You may feel irresistibly tired.*

- *If healing is being directed at a particular part of your body you may feel tingling, warmth, coolness, expansion, or a pushing sensation.*

- *You may notice the room appearing to change colour (probably the colour of your aura changing).*

- *You may find images coming into your mind or a flooding of an emotional reaction, especially tears or laughter, followed by a sense of relief.*

- *You may experience overwhelming love or joy.*

- *One of the most powerful healing experiences is a deep sense of surrender, perfection of the moment, and thankfulness for life.*

Powerful healers can generate intense brain-wave patterns... corresponding to brain states that are most conducive to healing.

relaxed, of putting the "normal" world into soft focus, and of accessing a profound experience of love, unity, or a personal vision of "God". This state is directed, with focused intent to heal, but without expectation of results, to the receiver. The intensity of brain-wave patterns seems to influence the client's brain waves to synchronize with theirs and it is this that probably stimulates healing. Colour changes in the aura seem to correspond to theta (blue) and delta (yellow) waves in the brain. This can often be seen as a tint to the vision. Many energy-healing techniques have a similar effect on brain waves, which may explain their effectiveness.

The other change in brain-wave pattern that seems to be involved in healing and in changes to the subtle bodies is the harmonization of the left and right sides of the brain. This can also be seen in the EEGs of healers and when people are being healed. Like brain waves this synchronization is transmitted from healer to client.

The left side of the brain seems to be the logical, intelligent, linear, and articulate part. The right side is the intuitive, feeling, creative part that deals in patterns rather than lines and thinks laterally. Humans usually work predominantly with one or the other side of the brain, and a balanced person can combine the workings of both. When the two parts are working synchronously, it appears to give us access to all our energy field and allows for healing to take place, as well as inspiration, intuition, and creativity of the highest order.

Many energy-healing techniques have the same effect of synchronizing the two halves of the brain that has been observed in healers. For most of us, who are left-brain dominant, creative activities will stimulate the right brain. Singing, playing music, and dance are particularly effective, especially if they engage the emotions, since they combine technical left-brain qualities with expressive right-brain qualities. Disciplines such as pranayama (see p. 92), tai chi (p. 84), and yoga (p. 82) can also develop this right-brain synchronization.

The jump from these changes in the brain to the effects on the subtle bodies has not been made by science, but it can be deduced by matching up objective evidence from scientific observations with subjective experiences. When healers describe what they feel in terms of changes in energy flow and in the subtle bodies, this consistently fits with the EEG changes observed by scientists.

OBJECTIVITY, SUBJECTIVITY, AND PERCEPTION

We perceive the world through our senses. Science has taken touch and vision and has built up a detailed understanding of the world based on what can be seen or touched and is therefore measurable. Sound, smell, and taste are measured in terms of touch and vision. Scientific perception, known as "objectivity", is based on measurement, and is considered to be free of personal bias that beliefs or preferences produce.

A view of the world, that includes personal biases, is known as "subjective". These biases influence how we perceive the world through our senses. They are subconscious and so influence perceptions without our being aware of them. These beliefs are formed by cultural heritage and personal experience, coloured by emotions.

Science dismisses subjective experience because it is aware of the distortion that emotion, belief, and preference produces. However the presumption that scientists can work purely objectively is naive. It is not possible to function as a normal human being without being subjective. This is how the brain works. The objective world of science is a theoretical non-real world, yet it tries to convince us that those things it can analyze and explain are real and those it cannot are illusion. A scientist is just as caught up in subjectivity as a mystic, probably more so, as the mystic practises internal ways of detaching from subjectivity. Meditation is a common way to achieve this. It is known that dowsers, healers, or psychics become inaccurate if personal preferences, beliefs, or emotions come into their work.

Right: Girl before a mirror, by Pablo Picasso

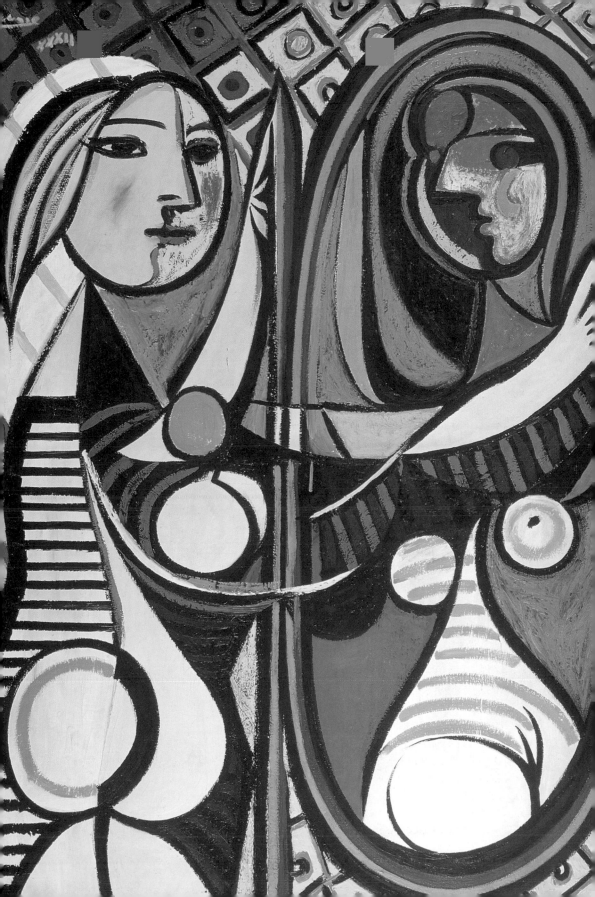

The problem with subjectivity is that much of it is based on unconscious, often negative, unevolved ways, of responding. This cannot be corrected by an increased reliance on science, but by renewing links with our mystical, spiritual life, that which science is taking such great pains to disprove.

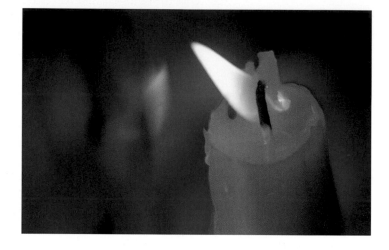

The increasing interest in energy healing is due not only to a disillusion-ment with medical science (not always justifiable) but also to an intuitive realization that false beliefs, chronic negative emotional responses, and lack of connection to something greater than ourselves lie behind the cause of much stress and disease.

We all work more or less effectively in our subjective worlds and rarely try to tackle true objective observation. If we did, every decision would take endless experimentation and analysis and even then would still be up for debate. We base decisions in all parts of our lives on subjective per-ception. This does involve physical observation, but much of our view of the observation is based on cul-tural values, past experiences, hopes and fears and, if we are fortunate, intuition. It is this subjectivity that gives our world its richness, excitement, mys-tery, and fulfilment. To consider this way of looking at the world wrong is to deny our human-ness.

...false beliefs, chronic negative emotional responses, and lack of connection to something greater than ourselves lie behind the cause of much stress and disease.

THE PHYSICS OF ENERGY

Physicists' attempts to explain how our world works have been influenced by new discoveries, from Newton's model of a mechanical universe 300 years ago, to Einstein's theory of relativity. Modern-day subatomic physics and quantum theory seem to be more in agreement with ancient mystical traditions of the interconnectedness of everything in the Universe. Over the next few pages we will look at how our theories and understanding of energy have developed.

ELECTROMAGNETIC ENERGIES

The meaning of energy

In the classical physics definition – energy as the capacity for doing work – work is the distance a force can move a body and a force is an external agency capable of altering a state of rest or motion in a body. In practical terms energy can be seen as the "strength" of a force.

When Newton (1642–1727) was studying gravity and defining the classical physics model, electricity and magnetism were seen as little more than curious natural phenomena. However by the 1800s, it was clear that they are forces capable of doing work and so are a kind of energy (see left).

Soon it was realized that these two energies combine to form a third range of energies which include heat and light. These energies radiate as waves and they all travel at the same speed – 300,000 metres (186,000 miles) per second, the speed of light. What differentiates the types of wave is their wavelength – for example infra-red radiation (heat) has longer wavelengths than visible light. We now know that the electromagnetic (EM) spectrum ranges from long wavelength, low frequency radio waves through microwaves, infra-red, visible light, and ultra-violet to higher frequency shorter wavelength X and gamma rays.

Two hundred years ago, when physicians started to investigate electricity and magnetism, it was discovered that these forces could be "seen", as they produced a whole pattern of force lines, now known as electrical or magnetic fields. Since the late 1800s such force fields surrounding living organisms have been measured. They are indicators to practitioners of energy healing that living organisms have a force field. But "life energy" cannot be explained by the theories of electricity and magnetism. However newer developments in physics theory provide explanations for energy healing that move beyond the need to explain it as an electromagnetic force field.

INTERCHANGEABILITY OF ENERGY AND MATTER

In classical Newtonian physics energy and matter are separate entities. Within this framework it is very difficult to see how energy can affect matter and therefore how healing using energy can affect the matter of the human body.

However, Einstein's General Theory of Relativity relates energy to matter. Einstein (1879–1955) developed his theory because he could not accept the Newtonian view that electromagnetic radiation waves must travel through a medium. As this medium could never be found it was hypothesized as being undetectable – "luminous aether".

Einstein tried unsuccessfully to detect luminous aether and eventually developed a theory to explain how light travels without this invisible medium. His Theory of Relativity postulated that if space and time were not absolute, but varied depending on the position from which they were being measured, the physics of light could be explained. Einstein had already worked out from his observations of light that its speed has the unusual property of being constant in all situations. Using this observation he also deduced that it moves at the fastest speed achievable by anything in the Universe. For his theory to work, time would have to be variable, depending on where it is measured from. Einstein's calculations predicted that time measured on an object travelling at high speeds passes more slowly than time measured on a stationary object. This has since been proved true.

As well as time passing slower and slower for an object as it travels faster and faster, Einstein's theory predicts that the object also gets heavier and therefore requires more energy to make it travel faster. Einstein worked out that as it approaches the speed of light it becomes so heavy that the energy required to move it faster would be impossible to provide.

For energy healing [Einstein's theory] is an especially interesting theory as its concepts appear to be remarkably similar to roots of Ancient Eastern philosophies as written in the Vedas.

Einstein's formula

In the formula $E = mc^2$, *E is energy, m is the mass, and c is the speed of light: 3.0×10^8 metres per second.*

The formula shows us that matter and energy are interchangeable. 1kg of mass is equivalent to $1 \times c^2 = 9.0 \times 10^{16}$ Joules of energy.

The only way to explain this would be for matter and energy to be related. By combining his Theory of Relativity with the old Newtonian theories of matter and energy he produced his famous $E = mc^2$ formula, which relates energy to matter (see left). Using this formula it can be shown that even the smallest particle, such as an atom, contains an enormous amount of energy. The atomic bomb has shown us that this matter can be exchanged and released as energy.

Einstein's theory of the equivalence of matter and energy has revolutionized scientific understanding of the world, especially at the submicroscopic level. For energy healing it is an especially interesting theory as its concepts appear to be remarkably similar to roots of Ancient Eastern philosophies as written in the Vedas. These consider that the material world is "condensed" out of a universal energy of which the cosmos is composed. These principles support theories of consciousness, psychic experiences, and the life force.

THEORIES OF ATOMIC STRUCTURE

The Ancient Greeks first developed the concept of the atom, but it was not incorporated into physics until the 1800s, when it was theoretically devised as being the smallest "whole" particle of matter. By the end of the nineteenth century the atom was proved to exist. Initially an atom was visualized as a minute ball which obeyed the laws of classical physics. But the discovery of the electron within the atom in 1895 opened up a whole new branch of physics – subatomic physics. Through the development of subatomic theory, assumptions about the structure of an atom have changed dramatically over the last hundred years. To date, an atom has been found to contain a plethora of component particles, for example protons, neutrons, and quarks.

With the discovery of the electron the structure of the atom was visualized as a "Christmas pudding", where the electrons were negatively charged "raisins" and the "pudding" was the positively

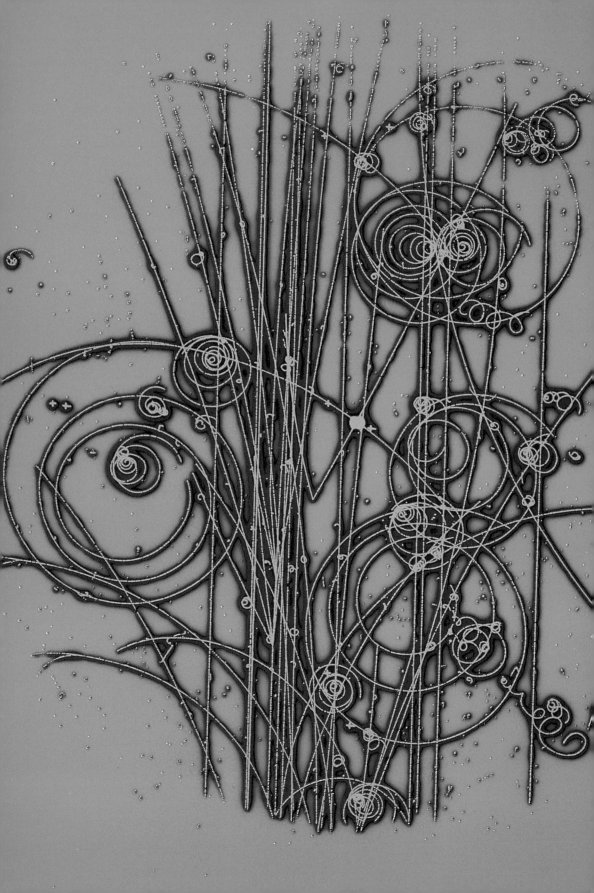

Wave/particle duality

In the 1900s quantum theory grew out of the inability of electromagnetism and classical physics to explain some experimental observations. For example, according to classical physics, since heat energy is a wave, some of the heat radiating from a fire would attain such a high frequency that it would set us on fire if we stood in front of it.

To explain why this does not happen it was deduced that electromagnetic energy is parcelled up into tiny units or packets of energy which behave like particles. These units are known as "quanta". Likewise visible light is made up of small units of energy called "photons".

Left: Tracks of subatomic particles in a bubble chamber, clearly showing the distinctive spiral paths of electrons and positrons.

charged matrix. However experiments soon showed that this model did not fit the facts and a new model gave a very different picture of how matter is built. Atoms were no longer considered solid but to be mainly space in which tiny particles, components of the atom, move at high speeds in fixed orbits. This model was devised by Niels Bohr (1885–1962) and is known as Bohr's atom. The theory needed to develop it is known as the "old quantum theory".

However physicists felt that there must be an explanation for why particles sometimes behaved like waves and sometimes like particles (see left). This grew into "new quantum theory", which suggested that this wave/particle dualism could be explained using probability. It is impossible to predict where exactly an electron might be at any time, but the probability of finding one in a given position can be predicted. This gave a new version of the atom – surrounding the nucleus is a "quantum" field that defines the area where the electrons surrounding the nucleus are most likely to be. This suggestion fitted the observations made about subatomic behaviour better than any other.

This theory also states that an electron behaves as a wave or a particle depending on the method used to detect it. Physics was now moving closer and closer to energy-healing ideas. For the first time in science it was recognized that the consciousness of the observer in the act of observing affects the outcome. An implication from this is that we observe what we set out to observe: consciousness becomes an influencing factor. This opens up the possibility that thought has an effect on what happens physically, making the energy-healing observation – that mind, consciousness, or thought can influence our physical selves – more scientifically acceptable.

Still quantum theory had facts that it could not explain. It had been found in wave/particle experiments that if two particles had been connected at one time they then remained connected in such a way that change in one seemed to be immediately reflected in the other. This instant transmission of information appeared to contradict Einstein's supposition that light travels at the fastest speed in the Universe. To explain this John S. Bell (1928–90) proposed an inequality theorem, which stated that in spite of what appears to be happening in our immediate surroundings, there is another, invisible, reality in which connection is always present and which allows for communication faster than light.

This progression of quantum theory brings science into line with the ideas of energy healing. Mystical tradition around the world considers that everything in the world is connected and many energy-healing practitioners use this concept to explain how energy used in healing can be effective and instantaneous, when supplied at a distance. As physicists are still debating whether this latest development of quantum theory is valid, so the scientific verification of this aspect of energy healing is still pending.

THE "FIFTH FIELD" OR QUANTUM VACUUM

The hypothesis that cause and effect may occur simultaneously, certainly at speeds faster than light, is now being seriously investigated. Scientists are proposing that, for this to be possible, everything must be interconnected.

This interconnection of all in time and space, while keeping this connection as a "memory", is again similar to esoteric teachings and would provide a "universal consciousness" capable of evolving the world. There is a scientific model that would allow for such a web to exist; the concept of the "hologram" (see right).

The idea of a force field analagous to the surface of the sea, which is capable of recording wave patterns in the same way as a hologram, has been suggested. It has been named the "fifth field" and said to lie beyond the space, time, matter, and energy concepts that physics normally deals with. It is theoretically thought to be the force from which the four other forces, or energies, of the Universe are derived.

If the underlying matrix of our Universe did indeed act like a hologram, a small part would

How a hologram is made

A laser beam is split and the two beams are passed through "diffusers", which produce many points of light. One beam is directed at the object to be hologrammed and the light bounces off it on to a photographic plate. The other beam is directed straight to the plate. When the two diffused beams reach the plate the interference pattern they make is photographed.

This holograph contains information about the surface of the object, which can be decoded by using another beam of laser light to view the plate. This reconstructs the object in 3-D form. The diffuse light used to produce the hologram repeats the interference pattern over the whole plate, so even a small part of it can be used to reconstruct the three-dimensional form of the object.

Virtual reality

In physics "virtual" means something exists, but not in measurable reality. Its presence can be deduced by extrapolating from information that is measurable. The image in a looking glass is a virtual reality.

Ocean waves

The waves on the surface of the ocean form two kinds of patterns. One is a steady form created by the coastline, and the other is a temporary form caused by passing boats. The steady form can be likened to the solid objects of our Universe and the temporary one to the electromagnetic waves that permeate it.

contain the information contained in all the rest of it, and so all parts would appear to be connected over time and distance. This holographic field could be considered the scientific equivalent of "God" in Judaeo-Christian tradition – "That which is now and ever shall be", and – "That in which I live and move and have my being", the Tao in Oriental tradition and Akasha in ayurvedic tradition.

For such a field to exist it would need a medium outside our concepts of space and time, beyond where the "probability fields" of quantum science and the "force fields" of classical science are known to operate. This medium has acquired the name "quantum vacuum". It has been postulated to exist, as physics has found a point where all traditional forms of energy appear to vanish, known as the "zero point". At this point a new set of "virtual" energies (see left) with properties that correspond to the measurable energies of the Universe appear.

The zero point seems to be the source of all the energy in our Universe. This idea has long been expressed in religions as "the void" or "chaos". In physics it is proposed that our physical Universe floats upon a "virtual" sea of energy that lies below or beyond the zero point. This is sometimes referred to as the "Dirac-sea", named after Paul Dirac, a great mathematician of the quantum era. Physics has been able to extricate some of this virtual energy into "real" particles, so there is some verification of its existence. It is possible that the explanation of matter "disappearing" into a black hole is that it enters this "sea" through the black hole.

Yet again these new ideas are changing concepts in physics that are as fundamental as mass, gravity, distance, and time. In the theory of the quantum vacuum, matter comes into existence when the "virtual" energy of the Dirac-sea interacts with electromagnetic waves to make holographic patterns on the Dirac-sea. The speed of these virtual energy waves has been calculated to be one billion times the speed of light, which is a contradiction of Einstein's observation that light is the fastest-travelling wave in the Universe. Most of the argument against the existence of subtle energies rests on scientists' inability to link these energies directly to measurable frequencies which travel no faster than the speed of light. Thus, once the possibility of such fast-travelling waves is accepted, much of the fabric of physics, that negates the existence of subtle bodies, subtle energies, and their ability to affect the progress of physical disease, crumbles.

For some time now science has considered that matter is composed of energy. This new theory proposes that there is a complex energy matrix underlying matter, without which the physical Universe could not exist. This theory does explain the Universe more fully than the theories that pre-ceded it, but as yet it cannot be detected with present-day scientific tools. This puts cutting-edge science in a similar position to ancient theories of energy healing.

Eventually science may become better able to understand the difficulties that energy-healing techniques have had in demonstrating subtle bodies. This may lead to more interest by scientists in these practices and possibly the development of more appropriate technology to detect and influence subtle energies and methods of healing.

Ancient religious texts such as the Upanishads of Hinduism and the Tao of Chinese philosophy are full of references that only become understandable today in the light of modern physics theory. For millennia mystics have described experiences of seeing the Universe in wave form. It is described as being made of light and the experience is of overwhelming bliss, joy, and love. Many healers describe the quality that they need to cultivate to promote their healing ability as love. This is the energy that seems to affect all the energy fields surrounding our bodies. Perhaps the fifth field is love.

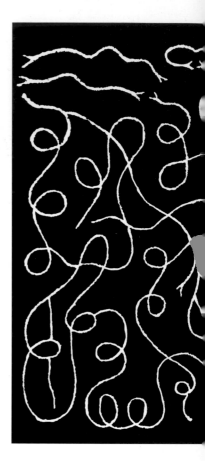

Ancient religious texts such as the Upanishads of Hinduism and the Tao of Chinese philosophy are full of references that only become understandable today in the light of modern physics theory.

TRADITIONAL VIEWS OF ENERGY

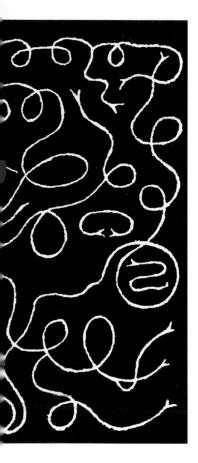

A representation of the penetrating force of the Vital Spirit and the links between the macrocosm and the microcosm, from the Taoist Canon, Tao-tsang.

According to classical physics life is impossible. The energy of the Universe, while it cannot be created or destroyed, is becoming redistributed so that high-energy states such as stars cool down, while the surrounding space warms up slightly. With this theory, the ultimate outcome of the Universe would be endless space containing star remnants, planets, and cosmic dust all at a uniform temperature and uniform energy level, which would be very low. This process of redistribution of energy to a overall lower level is known as "entropy".

However this physics takes no account of the living systems that exist on Earth. "Life" is able to reverse this process of entropy. It is able to create complex forms that can store energy.

There is obviously something special about living things that both classical physics and modern medicine (which is based upon it) ignore. However this attitude is only relatively recent. Ancient cultures acknowledged the presence of life and related it to health and wellbeing. This concept is known as "vitalism" and it is the opposite of entropy.

VITALISM

Energy-healing theories are based around the ancient concept of "vitalism" – a force that distinguishes living from dead forms. This energy, responsible for aliveness, health, and wellbeing, is known as chi, qi, or prana. Hippocrates (d.377 BCE) described it as the *medicatrix naturae*; Hahnemann (1755–1843), the founder of homeopathy, called it the "vital force". It is also known as "life force", "soul", "spirit", or "consciousness"in different traditions.

Classical physics would consider the process of life as the ability to decrease entropy. Modern physics might see vitalism as the culmination of the evolution of the complex wave/energy structure that is the Universe. This structure is evolving to accommodate more and more subtleties of which life, followed by conscious mind, seem to be the present end results. It would appear that life is a property of the fifth field (see p. 30).

This theory supports theories of energy healing. The subtle energy bodies (see pp. 36–40) that are so hard to find using scientific technology, could be formed of fifth field energy. This would also explain why electromagnetism is often considered part of the mechanism of energy healing, as both electromagnetism and matter seem to be generated in a similar way by this fifth field.

The holographic properties of the fifth field suggest that it could be the basis of thought and consciousness, explaining why these are important parts of energy-healing techniques, especially those using psychological methods.

CREATION THEORIES

Cosmology (how the world began) is similar in all major religions. Once these ideas were considered "truths", but the rise in influence of science has at least temporarily undermined them. However present-day science is now coming to the same conclusions as these religious traditions. Ancient philosophical thought considered that what happened on a grand scale in the cosmos was mirrored in what happened in our own surroundings and lives. The similarity of the outer Universe beyond the Earth and the "inner" universe at the subatomic level is a current example of this concept and an example of "as above so below" – the microcosm reflecting the macrocosm.

Western religions link closely to the ideas of alchemy. This "royal art" originated in Ancient Egypt and its ideas are found in Judaism, Christianity, and Islam. The Eastern traditions of Hinduism, Buddhism, and Taoism all link into a similar root, which stem from the Vedic texts of Sanskrit. It may be that the Vedic and alchemical traditions were in themselves also linked.

All these traditions see that there is a state before creation which contains everything, but as an

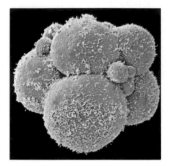

The microcosm in the macrocosm

The conception and development of the fetus mirrors the traditional views of creation. How life comes into being still cannot be explained by medical science.

The underlying source of everything seems to give the sperm and ova the potential for new life. When they come together they initially become one, but immediately start to divide again and again to form cells, as shown in the eight-celled human embryo, above. Initially there is no differentiation of the cells, equivalent to the unfolding of the energy of the Universe before it becomes recognizable as matter.

Eventually these dividing cells form a complete, separate organism that has a life of its own and is ready for birth into the world. This is the physical and subtle energy construct that we recognize as a living being.

indivisible unity. This state has always been present, is present now, and always will be. It is hard to comprehend this state, as we exist within it and can never reach its limits. Creation manifests when this One-ness moves and generates a duality, since the movement of one part of this One-ness necessitates a reaction from the rest of it. This duality is the basis for manifestation of something that we can begin to comprehend – energy, which ultimately "condenses" into physical matter. Mystics experience this energy as "light", it is chi or prana in Oriental traditions, and "quicksilver" or "mercury" in alchemy. It is the basic energy of the Universe and appears in different forms depending on what level it is being considered at. In terms of healing it is the life force, but in physical terms it is electricity.

The originators of this energy seem to be the opposite poles of creation. It is lightness and dark-ness, or male and female. In Taoist tradition it is yang and yin; in the Bible, heaven and earth; and in the Vedas, purusha and prakriti. Once this duality is created, subsequent steps instantaneously multiply it to produce the infinite complexity of the known physical world.

In many traditions, the elements are seen as manifesting from this original energy. There are four or five elements, depending on the tradition, but on closer inspection the four in some theories can be taken together to form a fifth. In alchemy the elements are earth, water, air, and fire, which com-bine to produce a fifth element: "quintessence" or "ether". In the Vedic tradition there are also five elements, with the same names and meanings as the alchemical elements. The Taoist tradition is a little different in that the fifth element is wood, not ether. Both Oriental traditions appear to miss out the stage of the four elements combining to form the fifth, but the roles the elements play in the development of the world as we know it is the same.

These elements should not be confused with their physical counterparts. Lack of real understanding of what these elements represent has cast a cynicism

...there is a state before creation which contains everything, but as an indivisible unity. This state has always been present, is present now, and always will be.

over alchemy and makes its Oriental counterparts difficult to understand. The elements describe an energy state, in the same way that water can be solid (ice), liquid (water), gaseous (steam). It is a way of relating what we perceive, from objects or emotions, to a place in the cosmos. From this understanding loss of equilibrium in ourselves preceding ill health can be seen as a loss of harmony between the elements that make up our being. Ayurvedic medicine and traditional Chinese medicine use these elements as tools for diagnosis and treatment.

Western medicine originally viewed illness in a similar way and the words "melancholic" (relating to earth), "choleric" (water), "sanguine" (fire), and "bilious" (air) are alchemical terms used to describe illness. Herbalism, the earliest form of "drug" treatment, was closely aligned to astrological indications, and astrology itself is closely linked to alchemy. Modern medicine is returning to these traditions in some branches of psychology; Jung (1865–1961) was a student of alchemy and saw how it linked into our imagination and thoughts.

Modern science, although it appears to differ from these teachings, has never explained the absolute origin of the cosmos. However the most progressive theories in physics are coming close to these ideas. Matter is now conceived as a form of energy which is the result of a merging of opposing forces, possibly the Dirac-sea and electromagnetic radiation. Behind all this is an inexplicable force – quantum vacuum (see page 30).

THE THEORY OF SUBTLE BODIES

One of the major pitfalls in the acceptance of energy medicine by today's scientific society is that it has been impossible to prove the existence of body energy using accepted scientific techniques. There is a lack of repeatability of test results and criticism of the scientific methods used constantly undermines attempts to prove the validity of energy medicine, in spite of the fact that these same problems are found in orthodox medical research.

However it is not necessary to use sophisticated technological techniques to detect body energy. Neither is it necessary to have psychic or mediumistic abilities. We experience this energy constantly, all the time. It is what activates our thoughts, emotions, and actions. It is the substance that gives us that quality we call "life". This life substance is like electricity in that when it flows through an appliance (or us) it (or ourselves) makes it work. And, like electricity, when it flows it creates an energy field. It is this that energy healers perceive surrounds and permeates the human body.

...[energy] is the substance that gives us that quality we call "life".

This body energy field or force field is often imagined as being made up of distinct layers, like an onion, but this is probably not accurate. Instead it seems to be a continuous band of energy vibrating at higher and higher frequencies. By looking at the body energy field frequencies Valerie Hunt, a medical scientist in the United States, has discovered that the frequencies become faster as the distance from the body increases. Even more remarkable, she has discovered that the predominant frequency in a person's energy field is the same as the frequency of the colour seen by reliable psychics. This ties up ancient teachings, psychic readings, and scientific observations in an astounding way.

There has been a long tradition of conceptually breaking down the body's energy field into different components. There are many similarities between these traditions. The Western tradition divides it into four main layers. The first is called the etheric, or health, aura. It is intimately connected to the physical body and appears to be a template around which the physical body is formed and maintained. This seems to be equivalent to the morphogenic field defined by Rupert Sheldrake and chi in the Chinese system. Acupuncture meridians are thought to be the link between the etheric and the physical body. These pass both over and through the physical body.

The etheric body is the one most easily seen in the "aura" by psychics. This body is closely linked to physical health and gives us our sense of aliveness

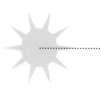

and wellbeing, or otherwise. It also forms our instinctual feelings – those that specifically protect us physically, such as "knowing" that a bridge is unsafe to walk on – as well as the reverse. Access to this information is more readily available to animals than to ourselves, as we tend to overlay messages from this level with our desires, fears, and beliefs, which arise in other layers of the energy field.

The second layer is the emotional, also known as the astral, body. This can separate from the etheric and physical bodies quite easily. Out-of-body experiences, shamanic journeying, and astral travel achieve this in order to travel in the universal, astral, or dream world realm as opposed to the physical realm. Every night we use this layer for dreams. The astral body constantly affects us during the day as well, as this is where most of our emotions originate. In our society many illnesses arise in the astral body due to our fascination with our emotions and our inability to handle them cleanly.

The third layer is the mental body. It is here that thought is generated. We can recognize this as our reasoning capacity. We have two types of thought and these are found in the mental body. The inner level is composed of concrete thoughts, such as when we plan a meal. Most of us spend a lot of time here and it is very tied in to our ego or personality. The higher or outer mental body is concerned with abstract ideas such as philosophy or theology. This outer layer contains our belief systems. Many of the beliefs we devise or have inherited are based on faulty or restricted reasoning and the untruth this generates is a source of much illness and unhappiness. Most of us are not consistently aware of this level of consciousness.

The fourth layer is the causal body, or higher self. This can be hard to access consciously, although it always supports and guides our other bodies. One of the purposes of spiritual practices such as meditation and prayer is to contact this layer consciously, in order to experience its support and guidance directly. It is this subtle body that receives

Enhancing awareness of the etheric body

The act of moving generates increased activity in the etheric body. This Sufi exercise formalizes the process:

1. Stand with your arms above your head and jump up and down. When you land, breathe out shouting "hoo!". Land hard on your heels. Keep this up as vigorously for as long as possible, then go on a little longer, before lying down.

2. Watch your body. Your breath is "breathing itself". You have temporarily released unconscious hold over natural breathing, freeing up energy flow. You will also be aware of your fast heart beat.

You may also notice other signs of trapped energy in the etheric and physical bodies (cramps, tingling, pain, numbness, or coldness), plus flowing, vibrating, warm, or expansive sensations – direct etheric body experiences. Sometimes the astral body is activated and you may feel emotions welling up. You may be lucky enough to access your causal body and receive visualizations, insight, and even the bliss of unconditional love.

WARNING: DO NOT DO THIS EXERCISE IF YOU ARE PREGNANT OR HAVE HEART DISEASE OR SEVERE ASTHMA.

the primary emotion, unconditional love. We experience this as the joy that seems to come from a welling-up or opening-up sensation in the heart area. Tapping in to this emotion is another benefit of spiritual practice.

If we receive information from the all-knowing source of the higher self, the understanding we experience is intuition. This differs from the instinctive information received from the etheric body in that it is based on all the conscious and unconscious knowledge we have, but is a leap beyond it. Once we receive intuition we can see with hindsight how we already had the information, but not the insight to make use of it. Everyone receives intuition in their own way. It might be an "obvious" realization after long pondering over a matter to no avail, or after a lot of thought a strong emotional drive arises to choose one course of action over others that may have made more logical sense. Often the information provided by the intuition very quickly proves itself to be the right decision.

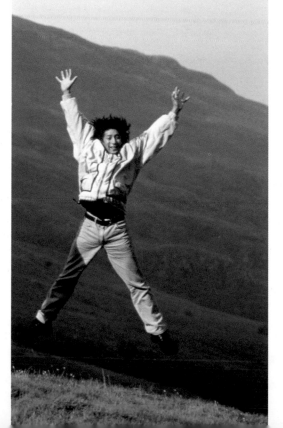

Following intuition

"I was on the brink of buying a holiday home. It seemed to have been provided by the Universe as my dream come true, but although I was very enthusiastic about it, I wasn't quite one hundred per cent sure. The night before I had to make my final decision I asked for guidance from my higher self and I awoke realizing the decision to buy would be foolish, as the project would use up much more of my time and energy than I had anticipated. I have never regretted the decision not to buy it as my intuition showed me that my time and energy is already spread quite thinly enough."

Helen

Our appreciation of body energy can be enhanced by practising exercises that increase conscious access to it. The main ways to achieve this are by movement, breathing, and visualization. For millennia esoteric traditions such as yoga, tai chi, chi kung, Buddhism, Sufism, quabbala, and alchemical practices have been using these methods for this purpose. Psychoactive drugs can also achieve this effect, but it is temporary, incomplete, and potentially damaging. Such drugs should be avoided for these reasons and also because they decrease rather than increase the natural ability to open up to body energies.

USING AFFIRMATIONS TO ACTIVATE ENERGY

Affirmations are an attempt to change behaviour and belief patterns that are causing us to be ill or creating other life problems. Belief patterns arise in the mental body and have a strong effect on the emotional body as they cause us to have distorted emotional responses. These can filter down to the physical body in the form of physical disease or psychological distress.

Affirmations influence the subconscious. They are positive statements, made in the present tense, that aim to change your health, lifestyle, or inner qualities to something that you desire, but do not yet have. Affirmations are invented in our waking, conscious minds, which, in spite of constant belief otherwise, can change very little. The idea then is to get the subconscious mind to accept the affirmation.

There are various ways to get the subconscious to accept the affirmation effectively. Firstly, wording is important. The subconscious does not work with words, but with images, feelings, body sensations, fears, and desires that words evoke. So wording must not include negatives as the subconscious will form an image of that negative, without taking into account the negation. If someone says "this will not hurt" your mind latches on to the word "hurt" and you expect pain, despite what you have been told.

The affirmation also needs to be made in the present tense, otherwise the subconscious will take

"Acting as if"
Affirmations are probably an adaptation of an ancient magical practice known as "acting as if", in which the desired quality is assumed to exist already and you live as if this were true. This practice is often done naturally and is part of how we learn as we grow up. "Let's pretend" games are an example. Acting out affirmations can be an excellent way of activating them, though this must be realistic. An asthmatic who stops taking medication as a way of acting as if he or she did not have asthma would obviously be behaving inappropriately, though changing habitual posture to that of a non-asthma sufferer would be of benefit. Methods such as Alexander technique can help in such cases.

How to make an affirmation effective

The way you present your affirmation is very important. Don't write it down hundreds of times, remember it every hour, or post it up everywhere. Like a truculent child the subconscious is bright and capable, but hates being nagged. It views this approach in the same way as commands and starts to ignore the affirmation.

Instead, help the subconscious accept the affirmation by tapping into its creative tendency. Write the affirmation in decorative script or illustrate it with drawings or cut-outs. Make a song or poem or dance to accompany it. This creates a sense of expansiveness, fun, and joy that the subconscious naturally responds to.

Asthma affirmation

If you have asthma you might use the affirmation, "I choose to breathe in and out with ease and freedom. I have all the air I need freely flowing in and out of me". These are not "true" statements, but this is how an affirmation works; what is desired has to be assumed to already exist.

the statement at face value and assume at some time in the future that this problem will need solving. So an affimation about asthma needs to be stated as "I can breathe freely and easily", rather than "I am going to be able to breathe freely and easily".

An affirmation should be phrased as a suggestion rather than as a command, which will irritate your subconscious because the affirmation is not – as yet – true. It is these very beliefs that have caused the problem in the first place, so they are already strong and will easily undermine your new way of being unless approached with care. So in the affirmation for asthma you would not say, "Lungs, breathe in and out freely", but rather, "I choose to breathe freely". What is important about an affirmation is the emotion you invest in it. Fear is undermining and is a common reason for failure, as this will reinforce negative beliefs. Desire is good as long as it does not become a craving. This is another way of expressing fear, that the positive outcome of the affirmation will not happen. Love is an extremely good emotion to carry the affirmation on.

Another way to increase the affirmation's access to the subconscious is to use it when the subconscious is more readily accessible to the conscious mind. Just before sleep and just after waking are good times. Using the affirmation during a period of relaxation, such as in an autogenic training session or a hypnosis session, are other, powerful ways.

There are two chief reasons why an affirmation fails. The first, where the negative emotional patterns that made the affirmation necessary in the first place become reinforced, should be overcome by performing the affirmation correctly. If you are still having a problem with saying something you feel is untrue, you probably need to look more deeply into the habit patterns or beliefs themselves.

The second common reason for an affirmation to fail is if it is being used to change something inappropriately. This is more difficult to overcome. Miracles do happen, but in the long term the use of affirmations to get what we want is not constructive.

We have all had experiences in getting what we want and then finding that we do not like it after all, or that it does not satisfy our needs. This is because our desire was originated in the emotional or mental body and did not come from the causal body. Indeed, in subtle body understanding a major cause of illness is not listening to this divine aspect of the self. The way to true healing is the realignment of the lower subtle bodies with this part of our being. Healing naturally follows. An affirmation that focuses specifically on this re-alignment is a type of prayer.

TRADITIONAL ORIENTAL MEDICINE

From traditional theories of cosmology (see page 34), Oriental sages developed a philosophy encompassing life energy, health, and illness, and from these a system of medicine. Probably influenced by the Hindu Vedas, the Taoist tradition of Chinese thought considers that everything in the Universe is created from energy termed "chi", with two fundamental forms – yin and yang – the duality basic to creation. Yang is usually termed the male principle and yin the female. However these definitions are too narrow. The two always stand for pairs of opposites, the yang describing the more active, hard, penetrating qualities and the yin the more receptive, soft, yielding qualities (see right).

Oriental philosophy believes that change is the only constant in the physical world, since the balance between yin and yang is always changing. This is easy to observe in nature, and the phenomenon of life. Nothing is entirely yin or yang. The well-known symbol of the "Tao" of yin and yang (see photo, right) shows two contrasting "commas" swirling within the enclosing circle. The points of contrasting colour within the commas remind us that within the yin lies the seed of yang and vice versa.

Everything has yin and yang components, and is relatively yin or yang to something else. For example, hardness is a yang quality and softness is yin. Diamond will write on glass because glass is yin

Right: The yang quality of fire and the yin quality of a cloud are combined in this 19th century Taoist weather manual.

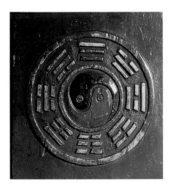

Examples of yang and yin pairs:
hard – soft
light – dark
positive – negative
male – female
convex – concave
warm – cold
sky – earth
fast – slow
focused – diffuse

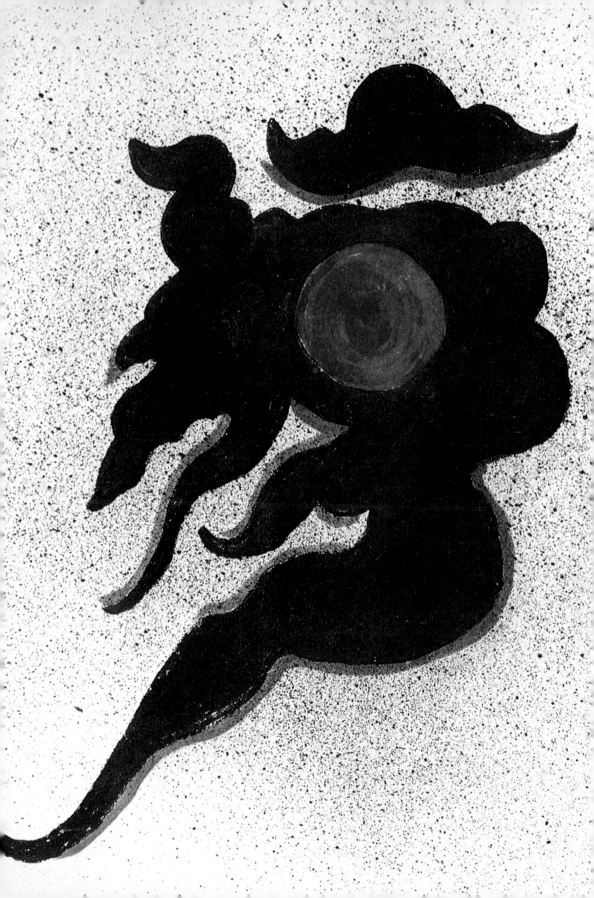

compared with diamond. But glass writes on perspex because glass is yang compared with perspex.

Chi is considered the basic life force and its flow is responsible for the day-to-day working of the living body and its protection against illness. Chi permeates the Universe. The formation of a human body fixes some of this chi in the life form and this is responsible for what we understand as life and health. Throughout life we continue to take chi in through food and breathing. The chi is distributed along invisible conduits known as "meridians". These pass chi along the surface of the body, where it protects it from disease attacking externally. Each meridian also flows internally, passing through the organ that it is named after. Within the body chi maintains a tension of life energy in the organ, somewhat similar to air in a car tyre, which enables it to function fully. The lines of the meridians also flow close to the nerves and blood supply.

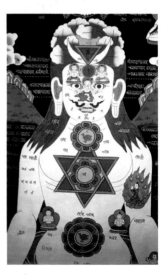

There are twelve bilateral meridians and two single, central meridians. They all run up and down the length of the body and are named after the organs to which they are related. The organs and their associated meridians form six pairs; within each pair one organ and meridian is considered to be yin and one yang. The two central meridians are the yin conception vessel (running down the front of the body) and the yang governing vessel (running up the back of the body). These meridians are not associated with any specific organs.

Oriental medicine has mapped points on the meridians, known as acupoints, where chi flow can be manipulated using needles or pressure. It has been suggested that the meridians lie at the junction between the etheric and the physical body and that the chi flowing along them affects the physical body by producing an electromagnetic field effect on the nerves and blood vessels that lie close to them. There does seem to be some electrical activity in the meridians. It has been shown that acupuncture points are areas of measurable decrease in the electrical resistance of the skin at this point. For a long

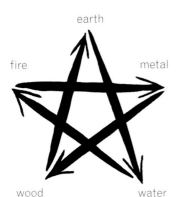

earth

fire   metal

wood   water

The two cycles

The five element theory consists of two basic cycles of rhythmic energy flow: the cycles of generation and destruction. In the cycle of generation chi flows from earth to metal to water to wood to fire and back to earth. This is often shown diagrammatically as a pentagon. The cycle of destruction connects the same elements moving from earth to water to fire to metal to wood and back to earth. In diagrams this is usually shown as a five-pointed star. So, if there is a build-up of chi in the wood element the treatment would be either to encourage more chi to move from wood to fire (using the cycle of generation) or to inhibit the flow into the wood element by emphasizing the element metal (using the cycle of destruction).

time the meridians were thought not to exist at a physical level, but to be useful as a map of energy flow in the body. However there has been scientific research that does support the physical existence of meridians.

Oriental medicine develops the idea of chi further. It postulates a more solid, slower-moving energy that contributes to the form and health constitution of the human body, known as "jing". Most of this is acquired from our parents at conception, but it can also be made from chi throughout life. The function of jing is to set the basic health constitution and to unfold the development of the body, from childhood, through adolescence to old age. It is particularly important in reproductive functioning.

The soul, or spirit, of the body in Chinese medicine is viewed as an integral part of the energy system of which the whole body is composed. This part of the energy system is termed "shen".

Five element theory

Oriental medicine uses another concept concerning chi flow to explain how the harmonious working of the body is maintained in health and becomes disrupted in disease. Once chi comes into physical form it flows through a cycle with five different qualities, known as the five elements. These are earth, metal, water, wood, and fire. Again, like yin and yang these are not literal subdivisions, but a way of dividing phenomena into five categories that is common to many ancient traditions. Chi in the body flows around the meridian system in a way that circulates it through these five elements. The organs and meridians are each associated with an element as well as having a yin or yang quality. For example, the kidney and bladder are water while the liver and gallbladder are wood.

If this natural flow is disturbed the balance between the elements is disturbed, which results in disease. The Oriental physician knows from the physical symptoms if the overall chi in the body is out of balance and also which element, or elements, are out of balance. He then applies his knowledge of yin and yang theory and five element theory to restore the level of chi and its free flow through the body. When these are corrected the chi goes on to influence the physical workings of the body and health is restored.

The correction of the chi can be achieved in several ways, often in combination. The most famous is acupuncture, but moxibustion, diet, herbs, chi promoting exercise (chi kung), and massage (tui na) are also used. Together these treatments compose the full spectrum of Traditional Chinese Medicine.

In both Chinese and Japanese cultures these theories of yin and yang and the five elements are applied to every aspect of living including food, environment, exercise (martial arts such as aikido and karate as well as tai chi), and lifestyle. There are also other methods of healing that draw upon these theories. Shiatsu (see p. 76) follows the tradition very closely and newer therapies, such as zero balancing (p. 91) and therapeutic touch (p. 80), have also drawn inspiration from the traditional Oriental system of healing.

THE CHAKRA SYSTEM

The Hindu religion has probably the most ancient sacred texts known, the Vedas, written in Sanskrit. These teachings describe a framework for the subtle anatomy of man that has influenced "New Age" thought more profoundly than has Oriental cosmology, though its source is often not realized.

This subtle anatomy and physiology cannot be observed in the detached way of science, but only by practising its existence. Then it becomes indisputably real. Prana is the basic life energy in yogic theory, corresponding closely with the Oriental concept of chi. This is what is meant by the term "energy" and is what we experience as being alive. This energy passes from the subtle bodies to the physical body via the chakras.

Chakra development, opening, or activation is a natural part of the evolution of a human being.

What the chakras mean

"Chakra" means "wheel" or lotus flower in Sanskrit (see right). Psychics see them as revolving (like wheels), coloured vortices of energy. The idea of the lotus flower comes from the fact that they are considered to have their roots in the physical body and flower in the subtle bodies. Depending on a person's stage of spiritual development the "flower" is either in bud, or partly or fully opened.

Each chakra is aligned to one of the major endocrine glands and also to a main nerve plexus in the physical body. It also relates to organs nearby. The seven chakras together cover all our activities; integration of the whole, thought, breath, circulation, digestion, reproduction, and excretion. They also relate to qualities of being; love, wisdom, radiance, assurance, realization, tranquillity, and patience.

Many other correspondences relate to the chakras, such as colours, gods and goddesses, sounds, and the astrological "personal" planets. The use of such correspondences enables better contact with chakra energy.

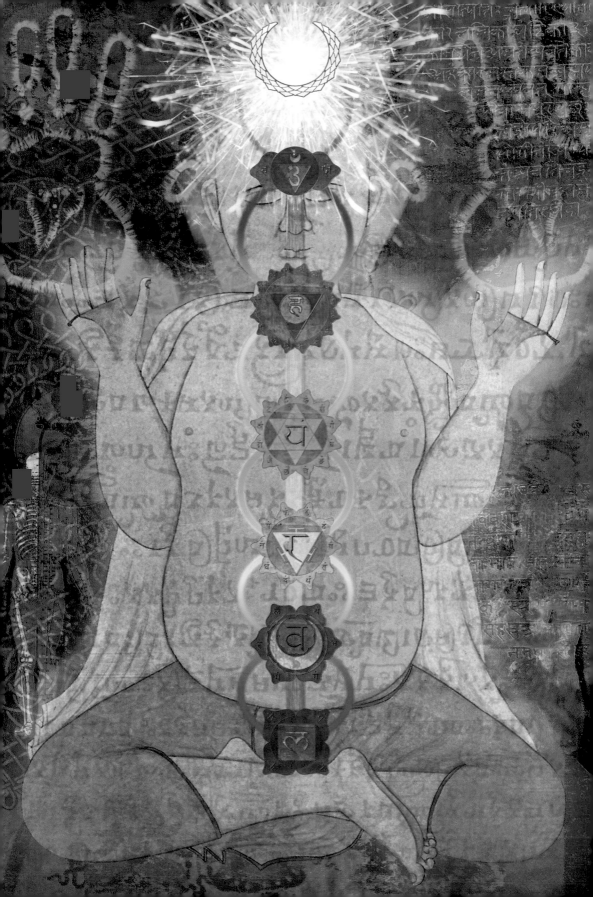

Working with a spiritual path in life encourages a speeding up of the activation. This happens in two ways. The first is more "Western" in that the development of the chakras is achieved by how we think and act in daily life. The "Eastern" approach uses this, but also uses physical and mental exercises to specifically activate the chakras. The first way is safest in the absence of a teacher because of the risk of activating the chakras inappropriately.

The chakras appear to be stepping-down points for the subtle prana from the Universe to enter the physical body. The close association between the endocrine glands and the nerve plexuses suggests that the activation passes to the physical through these anatomical structures. As both are essential for the harmonious functioning needed for the body to remain healthy, this is plausible.

Once the energy transmuted by the chakras interfaces with the physical body, it circulates through energy ducts known as "nadis". The Upanishads talk of 350,000 nadis, but there are fourteen main ones. It is interesting that there are also fourteen main meridians in Oriental medicine (see p. 44) and it is possible that the two concepts are related. By way of the nadis, every cell of the body is energetically connected to the whole.

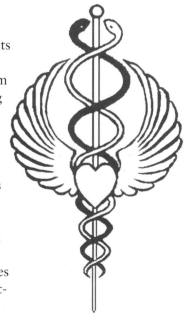

There are also two more, less well known, aspects of the Sanskrit subtle anatomy. The first is the sushumna nadi. This is an energy flow passing from the base of the spine to the top of the head, linking all the chakras from the crown to the base chakra. It is known as the "channel of fire" and is the most important nadi. The sushumna splits into three concentric forces. The innermost, citrini, balances the energies of the two outer forces and is known as the "heavenly way". The middle force is known as "vajra" and is an active, forceful energy, while the outer force is known as "sushumna" and carries inertia and inactivity.

It is along this nadi that the Kundalini energy rises if activated. Kundalini is the serpent goddess, depicted in traditional paintings coiled around the base chakra. When awakened she rises through the chakras, activating each in turn. Once Kundalini reaches the crown chakra, enlightenment is achieved.

This activation also affects the physical body, presumably because of the links between the chakras and the physical body. The experience is not to be viewed lightly. A great deal of caution is given in all teaching against forced activation of chakras, particularly by premature activation of Kundalini. The energy generated is too much if the physical body has not been properly prepared. This can lead to psychological and even physical illness or madness.

Interlaced with the sushumna nadi are two other forces, ida and pingali. The ida relates to the Moon energy, which suggests that it is "yin" in Oriental thought and the pingala is related to the Sun, which suggests that it is "yang". These two energies form an interlocking coil up the central column of sushumna. The pattern produced is remarkably like the wand of Hermes (see facing page) that Asclepias, the mythological father of medicine, traditionally carries. It is the same symbol used today to signify modern medicine.

...psychology, with its interest in the conscious and the subconscious mind, may influence the energy field of the individual, and hence the health and vice versa.

The ida and pingali energies relate to the chakras, though it is not clear if the chakras form the point of crossing of these two forces or if they form in the space between the points of crossing. The ida and pingali energies may be generated by, or themselves generate, the differing activities of the right and left sides of the brain. This might be a way in which psychology, with its interest in the conscious and the subconscious mind, may influence the energy field of the individual, and hence the health and vice versa.

Finally, Ancient Sanskrit teachings surround this framework of subtle anatomy with the four subtle bodies described on pages 36–40.

PERCEIVING ENERGY

Science has so far been unable to measure the subtle energies of the Earth or of the human energy field, which is why so many scientists are sceptical of their existence. However throughout the ages and in all cultures there have always been people who have been able to detect these subtle energies, through a "sixth sense" or mystic ability.

PERCEIVING THE AURA

The energy field surrounding the human body has traditionally been called the "aura". Most of us pick up emotional impressions and so are aware of the emotional aspect of the aura without being able to see or feel it. One dictionary definition of the word aura is the emotional impression made by a person or place. Sensitives can also see or feel the aura of people, places, or objects.

The aura is the energy field of the body and is made up of the subtle bodies (see pp. 36–40). At present, knowledge of the subtle energy fields, or aura, is largely subjective. Kirlian photography is one way of viewing the aura scientifically, but this and other methods designed to measure and record the aura have failed to gain scientific acceptance. Many of these techniques appear to be variations on dowsing (see pp. 52–4).

Everything in the Universe, whether inanimate or animate, has an energy field, since matter is itself a condensation of energy (see pp. 26–7). This field is the equivalent of the etheric field of the human body. In animate beings, emotions and thoughts add more layers to the energy or auric fields and compose the emotional and mental bodies. Thus the human aura is more complex than animal auras, and is also different from them in having the causal body, which relates to the higher self, or the "divine". All physical objects and animate beings are connected by their auric fields to the One-ness of the energy that is the Universe.

Seeing the aura

• *Stand your subject against a white wall in a dim light so that the body has a clear surround behind.*

• *Focus at the top of the head and then sweep your eyes around the body several times. Bring your focus back to the head and concentrate for about 15 seconds – then let your eyes go into soft focus.*

• *The aura usually appears first around the head and shoulders. Initially you may see an effect like a heat haze. White is usually the first colour to appear. Other colours may be fleeting, but with time and practice they will become more consistent.*

Feeling the aura

Stand behind your partner and rub your hands together for 30 seconds. Then hold your hands either side of the base of the skull, without touching. Spend time in this position to harmonize you and your partner's auras. Then move your hands around the space 10 to 15 cm (4 to 6 in) from the body. You may find it easier to keep one hand still and use the other to sense changes. The left hand is usually more receptive.

The areas corresponding to the chakras are easiest to detect. You may feel sensations of tingling, warmth, coldness, a "bulge", or a "hollow".

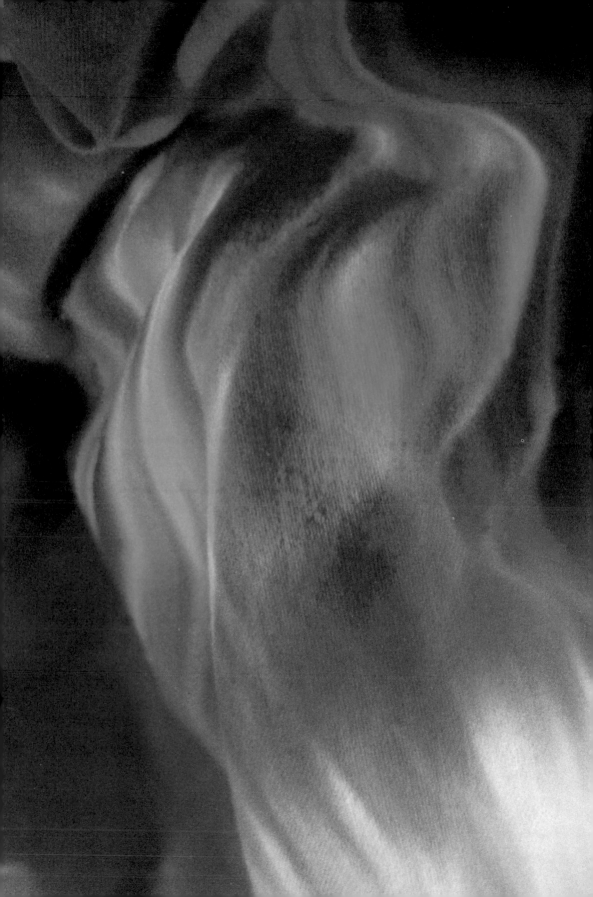

The size of the aura varies from person to person and from moment to moment. People with obvious vitality or charisma have larger auras. The aura may appear to extend for just a few centimetres (or inches) or up to several miles, as occurs with certain spiritual teachers. As people become more connected to their spirituality their auras extend and become more intense. Most of this extension seems to occur in the mental and causal bodies.

Most illness can be seen or felt in the etheric body, though it is often generated in the emotional and mental bodies. People who work with the auras, either in diagnosis or treatment, are interested in areas of the aura that feel disharmonious or look dull or damaged.

Intuiting the aura

Some people have a natural ability not actually to see or feel the aura but to intuitively know about it. This ability can take several forms. Some people feel the emotions of their subject, other people feel symptoms or pains, while others pick up images.

People with this type of ability often repress it. Without discipline or training a person can become overwhelmed by the suffering of others. However, with training these abilities can be developed to become an invaluable tool for diagnosis and treatment in energy healing.

THE THEORY OF DOWSING

Dowsing has always been considered magical, thus provoking scepticism. It is not a treatment, but an ancient tool for discovering information not directly available to us, probably from the etheric body.

All dowsing methods are based on the theory that subconsciously our bodies can detect changes in adjacent energy fields. Anything we come into contact with, whether in physical or energy form, creates a change in our field. Although this effect is mainly on the energetic or etheric body there are also small changes reflected in the physical body. These are thought to be electrical and cause small

Exercise

Rub your palms briskly together for about 30 seconds then hold your hands about 60 cm (2 ft) apart, palms facing. Keep your hands relaxed, but be aware of sensations. Bring your hands together slowly. Before they touch begin to draw them apart again to about 15cm (6 in). Do this several times. You will start to feel sensations that you previously had not noticed, often a sense of "sponginess". You are feeling the inner layers of your aura pushing against each other.

WARNING

• *Never look for or feel a person's aura without permission. This is an invasion of their privacy.*

• *Never "work with" a person's aura or energy field without permission. You cannot know what needs to be done. Subtle body healing is allowing energies to move as needed, not detecting what is wrong and fixing it.*

• *Never make the diagnosis of a physical illness. Accurate interpretation of an aura is complex and should be used only in conjunction with other information.*

• *Be careful whom you allow to contact your subtle bodies. Avoid those who want to "balance" or "open up" your chakras. This can disturb the natural unfolding of your spiritual consciousness.*

changes in muscle tone or in electrical resistance across the skin. All dowsing techniques work by amplifying these changes.

One of the popular uses of dowsing is in detecting water underground, since water, like all physical substances, has an energy field. Other examples of dowsing for environmental energies are discussed on page 56. Also dowsing can be used to obtain information about the human body. It is not clear how dowsers do this, but it is likely that they tap into the client's etheric body via their own.

Dowsing becomes complicated and less accurate than basic theory would suggest because the etheric body is also affected by changes in the mental or emotional bodies. This means that beliefs, thoughts, and emotions can all influence dowsing, which easily falsifies results unless the practitioner is skilled at keeping the mind clear. Clients, too, can influence dowsing in this way, although they usually have less ability to do so. It has proved difficult to investigate dowsing scientifically since the act of observation may influence the dowsing in the same way, producing incorrect results.

Dowsers can work without picking up on their own problems because they focus on the patient, using energy changes in their own energy field to perceive changes in the patient. Sometimes a practitioner works with a sample from the patient, known as a "witness" (see p. 54). This can be blood, hair, or even a signature or photograph. It appears that changes in the patient's energy field are passed on to anything that can be identified with the patient. Even more extraordinary, changes in the patient's energy field are constantly reflected in that of the witness. This means that the same witness can be used indefinitely as its energy field constantly adjusts to the present state of the patient. This ties in with the modern scientific proposition that everything is interconnected via the fifth field (see p. 30).

Some dowsers will ask for no additional information apart from a witness, but others will incorporate dowsing into a discussion of your

Dowsing methods

There are many methods of dowsing. The use of a forked hazel twig or a pendulum are the most traditional. Another common method is to use two L-shaped pieces of wire held loosely in the hands.

There are also highly sophisticated methods that use "machines" such as Radionics and the Vegatest. In Radionics, practitioners use a witness (see p. 54) in the apparatus (often known as a "black box") to detect what is wrong and also to transmit radionic treatment to the patient. The Vegatest machine measures changes in electric potential across the skin to diagnose areas of weakness and also the homeopathic remedies needed to balance the system.

Another recent extension of the dowsing principle has been the development of muscle testing, or applied kinesiology (see p. 77).

problems. When a dowser wants to discover a whole range of information, for example in checking for food sensitivities or suitable medications, different samples of the substances to be checked are held against the body or in the mouth. These samples are also known as witnesses.

Other dowsers do not use witnesses. They rely entirely on their ability to concentrate thought on the specific information they want. Thought itself creates an energy field change in the mental body and this filters down to the etheric and physical bodies, so this method is perfectly valid.

Some practitioners use dowsing to diagnose what is wrong, physically, emotionally, or even spiritually, but this requires penetration further into the subtleties of the client's energy fields and thus increases risks of inaccuracy. Also using dowsing at other levels of subtle bodies can develop a tendency to rely too much on the technique, which can become misleading and inappropriate.

It is easy to learn dowsing yourself. Everybody has a natural ability, but open-mindedness and practice will greatly enhance it. Initial experiments are usually uncannily accurate. However, with time, pitfalls become apparent. For example dowsing develops the power of the mind to influence the results, so that you may find that you start to pick up what you are expecting to find, rather than what is actually there.

EARTH ENERGIES AND HEALTH

The Earth is a living organism, with animals, plants, and humans living symbiotically. It has a complex energy body, which interacts with our own subtle bodies. The Earth's magnetic field, gravity, and the Aurora Borealis are the most physical manifestations of its energies, and are easily scientifically detectable, but there is a whole range of subtle energies present on, in, and above the Earth. Ancient civilizations, highly attuned to these, located sacred buildings so that building and Earth energy could work together. They knew which areas to avoid and how to divert

How a witness might work

One of the most difficult aspects of dowsing to comprehend is how a picture, map, sample of writing, or even a thought can work instead of the actual person or substance. Dowsing seems to work with the body-mind or subconscious, probably represented by the etheric body. There seem to be many similarities between the workings of this and the conscious mind.

If you see a real apple you understand what it is. If you are shown a picture of an apple, it is just as easy to understand what you are seeing. If you see the word "apple" you still understand what is referred to. If you hear the word "apple" you also understand it. If you think of an apple you know what you are thinking about. All these representations are physically very different. However the mind can tell that they all represent apple, perceiving the essence (spirit or energy) of apple which is transmitted in different ways by different physical mediums. It is this essence that is transmitted by a witness.

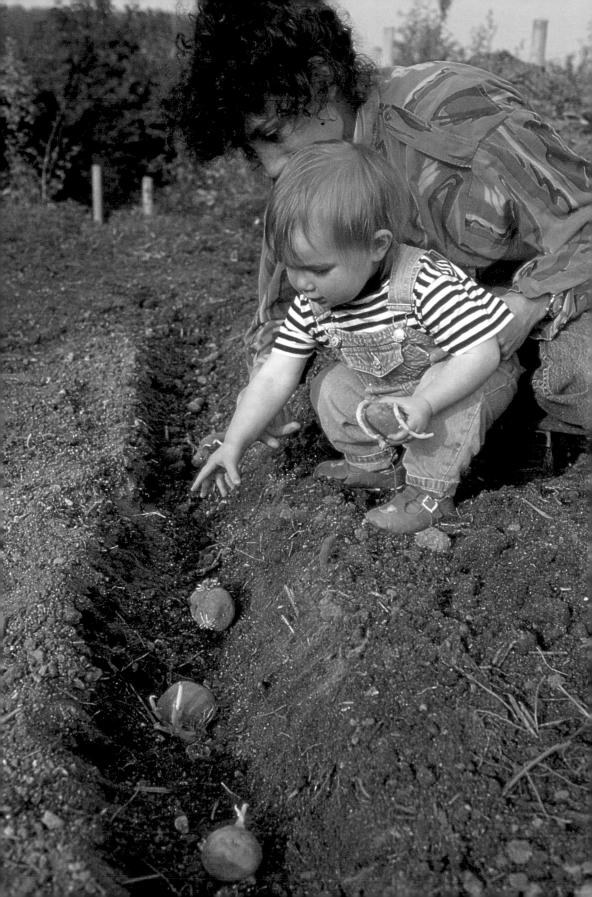

difficult energies; some ancient standing stones may be evidence of this.

Modern society has lost the sensitivity to these energies. We build homes, towns, and cities without bearing any of this in mind, and some materials and settings may even be physically or energetically harmful. This loss of connection with planet energies, and how this relates to its physical as well as its subtle nature, facilitates ill health.

An obvious example of our lack of connection with the Earth's energies is the way in which we disregard weather and seasons. We eat out-of-season foods, centrally heat and air-condition our homes, and use artificial light. This makes it hard for our physical and subtle bodies to keep in tune with the planet's natural cycles. Being in alignment with these cycles is healing in itself and disregarding them leaves us vulnerable to disease.

We can restore harmony between ourselves and the Earth by becoming aware of where and how we live. We can use locally available and natural building materials. Dowsing can be used to detect geopathic stress – areas where the Earth's energy is disturbed, for example by electromagnetic fields or underground water flows. We can also become more aware of weather and the seasons, spend time outdoors, and eat local and seasonal foods. These activities have physical and subtle body effects, especially on the etheric and emotional bodies.

The other aspect of the cycles of the Earth that we have become distanced from is patience, or waiting for the time to be right for change. This is a contented waiting, not a bridled anticipation; the body has a tremendous capacity to heal, but it takes time. Slowing down and becoming conscious of the time needed is a major step, as is becoming aware of the supportive and healing aspects of the Earth itself.

INTERPERSONAL ENERGIES

To a great extent it is the effect of our own energy fields upon other people's that determines their response to us. Although much of our impression of

Home and health

The home can enhance health or create dis-ease. If a home is placed well, made with natural materials, and lived in by a loving family, it will be an invaluable source of revitalization and healing. Even if these features are lacking, working with geopathic stress, redecoration and re-organization of space, and creating joyful family rituals, can create a healing environment.

The home should be both physically comfortable and visually appealing. Clutter should especially be avoided. There should be communal and private space to let relationships ebb and flow. There should also be "sacred space", a quiet room containing reminders of that which you hold dear or sacred (family photos, travel souvenirs, or found objects). In some religions, artefacts, or even small shrines – for example crucifixes, statues, icons, or altars – are an essential part of the home.

someone is based on looks, dress, speech styles, and the situation, the emotional attraction or repulsion is a direct energy-field interaction. We can view interactions between people as akin to two complex magnetic fields coming together. Some areas attract and feel harmonious, some repel and create tension, while some are neutral. Astrology can map out this interpersonal field and detect areas of harmony and conflict between individuals. This interaction is known as "synastry" and is a means of objectifying these experiences.

When there are attracting fields between ourselves and another person we tend naturally to trust, enjoy, and be open with each other. At its most intense this is falling in love, which leaves us most open to healing from the Universe. Cultivating this state by consciously enhancing feelings of attraction toward others is a wonderful way of both enhancing your own healing and that of others. To achieve this we have to release trapped and distorting emotional patterns, and inappropriate or faulty beliefs. This can be done by working with psychological tools, but it can also happen "by the grace of God", when we open ourselves to what lies beyond emotional and mental realms.

However, when we feel antagonism toward another this does not necessarily mean that our energies are inherently incompatible. With effort these energies can be transformed. Antagonism usually suggests that two people have not developed their capacity to see beyond personal viewpoints, or else they trigger each other's emotionally weak or distorted areas. Both are distortions in the subtle energy fields. Both people experience a healing if these distortions can be seen and released and the level of trust and openness can begin to increase. Normally both people contribute to the distortion. Each interaction we have is an opportunity to refine our ability to achieve harmony with ourselves and others. Healing of our relationships and our personal inner destructive patterns that can lead or contribute to illness automatically follows.

Showing our energy field

Physical attributes are how we physically advertise our energy field. Details such as the clearness of eyes and skin, and the condition of hair, reflect not only our state of health but also our emotional state, our belief patterns, and even our level of contact with the "divine".

THE SIXTH SENSE – EXTRA-SENSORY PERCEPTION

This is the ability to perceive something that is not physically apparent – a vision, a sensation, or words, and occasionally a smell or a taste. It may also come into the mind from no apparent source – often called "intuition".

Sixth sense is often associated with the ability to see or feel a person's energy field, or aura, and is sometimes associated with sensing what is wrong with someone, or the ability to feel another's symptoms or emotions. It is usually associated with an ability to heal. There are other examples of sixth sense, such as seeing the future, or what is going on elsewhere, or "reading" thoughts.

For millennia people have been interested in this sensitivity. It generally produces intrigue, fear, or scepticism. Recently scientists have been investigating claims, but so far data has not proved anything conclusively. There are reasons for this. To begin with there are hoaxers, who undermine belief that other cases may be genuine. Also true sixth sense tends to be unpredictable, which encourages disbelief. Using the sixth sense is rather like fishing in the Dirac-sea – the universal consciousness, or "memory", of all existence (see p. 31). You may bait your line correctly, but this does not mean that a fish will bite.

Interpretation can also be a problem. Extra-sensory information has to be interpreted by the mind and is more open to misinterpretation than things we can physically see, touch, or hear. This also makes experiments hard to verify, as a sensitive may not be able to pick up information so readily if the experiment is repeated.

Another problem is that scientists do not realize how much their own thoughts and feelings influence experiments. They are good at eliminating external clues and recording brain-wave patterns, but are not so aware of how their own thoughts and ways of measuring results influence the situation. This is an area that the cutting edge of modern physics has also found to be a problem (see p. 26).

Entrainment

Extra-sensory phenomena seem to involve changes in brain waves, the same way as in healing (see p. 20). When these phenomena occur the brain waves seem to switch to different frequencies, and if two people are involved the two brain-wave patterns tend to become similar. This is known as "entrainment".

The alpha, theta, and delta waves seem to be involved. Theta waves are mainly seen in healing situations, and the very slow delta waves seem to be necessary for distance work, such as sending information from one person to another, or "seeing" what is going on at a different location. It is possible that these waves are an indication that the human consciousness is tapping into levels of reality beyond the physical. These areas are now being explored by modern physics, where they are explained as the "quantum vacuum" or Dirac-sea.

WARNING

The use of sixth sense to contact the dead is to be avoided as this can cause serious psychological problems.

Extra-sensory perception can be developed just like any other skill. Spiritual healing trainings include this as part of the development of healing ability.

MIRACLES, LOVE, THE DIVINE, AND SURRENDER

Energy healing incorporates all methods of healing, from the orthodox "mechanical" approaches of drugs and surgery, to complementary therapies that enhance the body's own innate healing processes. Both these approaches affect the body's energy fields. In addition, energy healing connects directly to the causal body, the "spirit", or "soul". This is the primary aim of some complementary "treatments" (two examples are therapeutic touch (see p. 80) and spiritual healing (p. 79)). But any therapy has the potential to help us increase awareness of this level, and with this comes the inherent healing ability to perform "miracles".

Unfortunately, accessing this degree of contact with our most subtle energy levels is unpredictable. Its occurrence seems to be "by the grace of God". The doorway to this level becomes available when we give or receive unconditional love. This loving has no conditions for acceptance, it is free of fear of rejection, and has no expectation of reward or reciprocity. It comes from beyond ourselves and is as though we both give and receive at the same time. To experience this we need to learn the true nature of surrender – surrendering to something more than we already know and understand. Approaching this can feel frightening, which may prevent us moving to the place beyond – a place of love and profound fearlessness.

Preparing for "miracles"

Meditation and spiritual practices can prepare us for "miracles". Hands-on healings can also aid preparation, as can psychological techniques that allow us to see deeper into our mental and emotional selves.

Creativity is another way of opening up to healing at this level. Writing, painting, music, dance, and performance – especially when improvisational – all open up spontaneity and celebration that can lead to accessing healing from the highest level.

Enjoyable outdoor activities can also allow us to let go of our mental and emotional selves and open us to the deepest parts of our being, helping us access healing from the highest level. Any activity invoking this sense of surrender of the Self, especially if it stimulates spontaneity and fills us with thankfulness, can open us up to the experience of the "grace of God" – healing from the highest level.

Part 2
Complementary therapies

Most illnesses begin as a disturbance in the subtle energy field, which envelops the body. Approaching illness at the energy level is a very effective way of promoting complete and long-lasting healing. Part Two takes the author's personal selection of 45 therapies from the wide range of treatments that work with these subtle energies. Each entry, based on in-depth interviews, explains the technique and describes how it might work, giving you insight into which therapies might suit you best. The therapies have been divided into 14 classes, according to how they access the subtle bodies to promote healing.

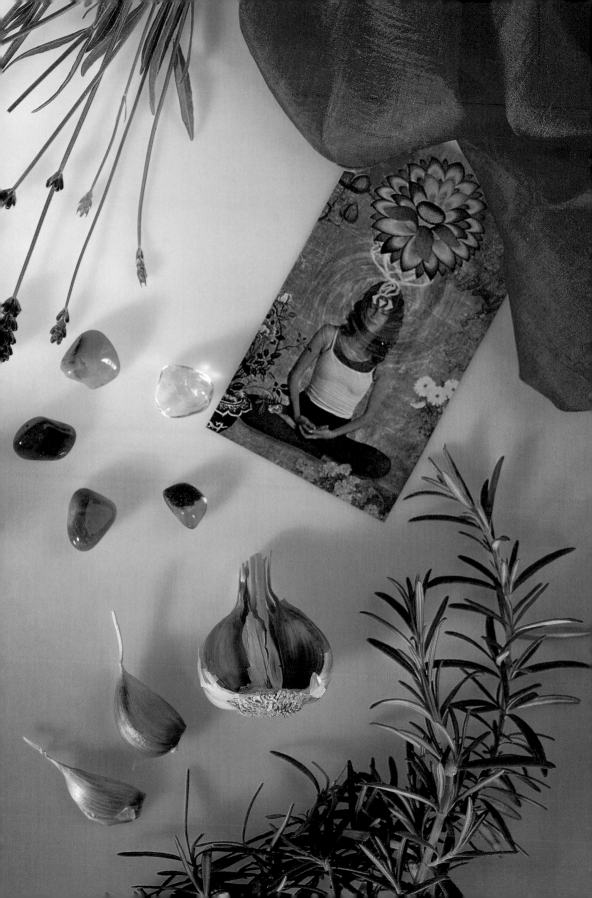

HOW TO CHOOSE A THERAPY

This book will give you a greater insight into your physical and energy bodies and also give you specific information on a wide range of healing methods. The charts in Part Three (see pp. 120–83) can give you further help in discovering where your major energy stumbling blocks are that prevent you from getting well. This information will guide you to the best therapies to try.

Self-empowerment is a major part of the healing process and any steps you make to take charge of your own healing are in themselves of great benefit. Once you have gathered the factual information, allow your intuition to draw you to a therapy that feels "good" to you. This may be a feeling of excitement, or the therapy may seem supportive. Or you may feel a fearful attraction that the therapy will draw you to an unknown that holds a key to your healing.

After deciding on a therapy the next task is to find a therapist. The best methods are by word of mouth, or by "synchronicity" – someone suitable "just happens" to come to your attention. If you can, speak to the therapist before you commit yourself, so that you can establish a rapport between you. Without empathy it is difficult to find the trust you need to enable you to surrender yourself completely to a new process of healing. You should choose an orthodox doctor in the same way. Empathy and trust in the relationship will allow subtle healing to take place alongside orthodox treatments.

Finally, it is important that you are comfortable with the costs involved. An expensive therapist is not necessarily the best person for you. But also beware of choosing a therapist because of their "good value". You are paying for the therapist's time, expertise, and premises. You can't buy or bargain a "cure".

...allow your intuition to draw you to a therapy that feels "good" to you.

THE ORTHODOX DOCTOR–PATIENT RELATIONSHIP

A good relationship between you and your orthodox doctor is important. Fortunately, increasing numbers of doctors recognize that treating the whole person is the best approach to healing. This is "holistic medicine", even though it is not using energy-based or complementary treatments. If your doctor is not this way inclined, or is not supportive of your interest in energy medicine, consider finding one who is.

The rapport you build with your doctor brings trust and openness, enhancing your natural healing mechanisms, which are what will ultimately overcome your disease anyway. More doctors are becoming receptive to energy-healing methods and your interest may well stimulate theirs. Some doctors welcome an opportunity for their patients to find a new way to health. However many are still sceptical. In some cases this may spring from a genuine concern for their patients' wellbeing, coupled with their own negative ideas or experiences of energy medicine. Sometimes a patient's decision to stop orthodox treatment for a scientifically untried energy-healing method may seriously jeopardize his or her health (terminating, for example, steroid tablets). Such treatments need to be monitored closely by a supportive medical practitioner.

Doctors are sometimes antagonistic about the use of complementary therapies when an illness is life-threatening and incurable, or when the treatment has only a small chance of being successful. Cancer and AIDS are good examples. Diagnoses of chronic and untreatable illnesses that can lead to severe handicap, such as multiple sclerosis, may also lead people to try alternative forms of treatment.

A person given a diagnosis of this type may feel let down by the medical profession and be willing to turn to anything rather than give in to a terminal diagnosis. Here orthodox doctors may feel helpless that they cannot offer a cure, but be unable to see that energy healing offers any better chance. Doctors are often also concerned that patients may spend money that they can ill afford receiving useless treatments. Ultimately the decision on whether to use energy-healing methods is the patient's, but this decision should not be made from a place of fear.

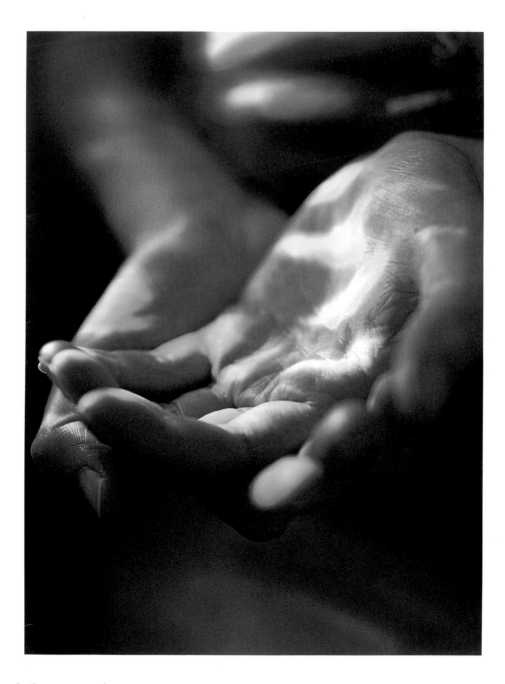

...subtle energies...
lie beyond everyday
understanding of the physical world.

IF IT'S SO GOOD WHY DOESN'T IT ALWAYS WORK?

In theory, every energy-healing therapy should be capable of curing every illness and relieving all our psychological distresses. Some therapists seem to believe that this is indeed so, but in reality it is not.

Scientists explain the failure of energy healing simply – it does not work. Successes are due to the placebo effect, "spontaneous" recovery, or remission. This can be valid for self-limiting diseases such as colds and 'flu, but not for illnesses such as cancer. Scientists also have difficulty accepting energy healing because the energies involved cannot be seen or measured. Some energy healers use scientifically based techniques to try to prove the existence of these energies. These may convince the lay public, but often scientists reject the methods for valid scientific reasons. Unfortunately both scientists and energy healers fail to appreciate that the subtle energies are likely to lie beyond everyday understanding of the physical world. Modern physics can supply an explanation, but physics theory at this level is also hard to prove.

There are also psychological reasons as to why treatments fail; both orthodox and energy medicine recognize this. Psychologically based explanations for illness consider that all disease arises from problems with emotions or beliefs. Thus a treatment may fail because of an unconscious desire to remain ill or an unwillingness to deal with emotional issues. For some this may be so, but it is not universal. The danger is that this attitude may undermine already low self-esteem and feed guilt. As self-empowerment and a deep sense of being loved are critical in healing, anything that destroys these may do more harm than good.

Failure to recover may also be because a person may believe that their body is incapable of healing itself, or that there is nothing in life worth getting well for. Such beliefs tie in with the emotions and also interfere with connection to the "divine". Changing beliefs is usually much harder than working with emotions. Sometimes it happens "by the grace of God". Miraculous healings seem connected with changes in belief, where the power of focused and consistent thought can have a very strong effect on healing. It is impossible to say how much illness is due to these psychological causes. However many people with serious emotional problems or inappropriate beliefs do not become ill, so this can only be a partial explanation.

There are also esoteric reasons for why people do not respond to treatment. Illness can be viewed as one of our greatest challenges – confronting us with mortality. Most spiritual teachings perceive that the maturing of our emotional selves and the emergence of our spirituality is greatly enhanced by illness. Healing often arises once life is stripped of its trivia and a person accepts what is really important in life and releases distractions. Also, healing does not necessarily mean restoration to good health. We must all die and for most of us illness is the gateway to death. Healing at this time, while not achieving a "cure", helps the person reach the end with deep love, completeness, and contentment.

In a very practical way energy healing has more difficulties interacting with the physical body than orthodox medicine. It is easiest and most predictable to affect the physical with the physical. This is true even though there is much evidence to suggest that our physical world is a condensation of energy and remains influenced by the energy world (see p. 26). One day we may develop tools that can forge a more predictable link between the energy and the physical bodies; however at present the best tool is another human. To enhance this link we need to shift our consciousness away from distractions and move into a "healing" state of mind. Just as a baby does not walk before its legs are strong enough, perhaps we cannot perform energy healing because we are not yet ready. The self-healing powers that yogis develop may indicate what is possible.

Finally, if healing does not occur, there is always the possibility that a chosen healer is insufficiently skilled, or the therapy chosen is inappropriate.

A mass leap of consciousness
Some spiritually based groups, such as the practitioners of transcendental meditation, believe that if sufficient numbers of people (often quoted as 144,000) attained a high level of spiritual awakening, humanity, as a whole, would make an evolutionary leap of consciousness. One of the benefits might be the ability to heal via the energy bodies, which might radically alter the effect of illness in our lives.

If your chosen therapy fails to benefit your health problem, look at the charts in Part Three (see pp. 120–83) to help you make a constructive and informed choice about the most suitable therapies.

DIET AND SUPPLEMENTS

Supplements

Food supplements are often used in conjunction with energy medicine treatments. The choice of supplements can be made in a number of ways. Firstly empirical knowledge of your illness may suggest a range of useful nutrients. Secondly question- naires or discussion of lifestyle, diet, personality type, and minor symptoms, as well as your illness, can help decide which supple- ments may be required. Thirdly blood or hair tests can be done to test for defi- ciencies. Finally dowsing techniques are sometimes used to choose supplements.

Unlike diet, supplements do not form a natural alliance with energy-based healing. The majority of them are produced in factories and bear little resemblance to the natural equivalent foods. They do not have the life force of fresh food. However they can interact with the physical body and so improve functioning. Then the subtle energy part of the being can function better.

The use of supplements is a "kick-start" to boost nutrient levels, while the rest of the treatment improves both the diet and the body's natural ability to make the most of its food. This is its valuable role as an adjunct to energy- based healing.

Diet plays an important role in many energy-based therapies. There are three major focuses of dietary approach in complementary medicine. The first is related to Traditional Chinese Medicine, the second to ayurvedic medicine, and the third to naturopathy and Western-originated systems of energy medicine.

All three approaches consider that an appropriate diet is necessary for wellbeing and that we are unable to cope with dietary stress in illness. Diet can be a tool to aid return to health – so illness demands a stricter diet than health does. All three also recog- nize that food carries "life force". Foods have herbal or therapeutic, as well as nutritional qualities. Conversely each system recognizes that some foods are bad for certain conditions or certain people.

Each system has a different way of selecting a diet to suit individuals and illnesses. For example, TCM classifies foods according to yin or yang and their affinity to the five elements. Ayurveda classifies foods according to the effect they have on the doshas, while the naturopathic system looks at food in a variety of ways such as its micronutrient properties, its detoxifying properties, its ability to provide life force, and its tendency to cause allergies.

The physical effect of diet influences our subtle bodies – they cannot function normally if diet is unsuitable. Other aspects of foods, such as freshness, rawness, organic growth, food combinations, amounts, place of growth, colour, texture, taste, cooking methods, source, time of day or season, and the love that has gone into preparation, all have effects on the way foods affect the subtle bodies.

Unfortunately the different dietary systems used in conjunction with energy healing do not necessarily agree. For example, a Chinese medical diet is likely to exclude dairy, while an ayurvedic diet may include it. And a naturopathic diet stresses raw food, while Oriental systems generally prefer cooked foods. This can be confusing if you work with more than one therapy. It is best to stick to one system and follow the guidelines of the therapist you have chosen.

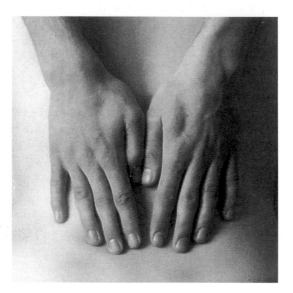

CLASS 1
Primarily physical techniques

massage
aromatherapy
osteopathy
chiropractic
Rolfing®

Methods that use touch or movement directly to affect the muscles, bones, and tissues of the physical body. At the same time they access the etheric body and facilitate changes in the emotional body. They also provide an opportunity for relaxation at all these levels.

Swedish massage

Most practitioners of Western-style massage base their technique on Swedish massage, developed in the 1700s by Per Henrick Ling. This system incorporates four basic actions:

PERCUSSION – *Using the side of the hand in a brisk, drumming movement.*

EFFLEURAGE – *Long, flowing strokes, using all parts of the hand, with either gentle or deep pressure.*

PETRISSAGE – *Kneading the skin. Used only on loose skin, such as the stomach.*

FROTTAGE – *Small circular movements using the fingers or part of the hand. Done at a light or deep level.*

MASSAGE

One of the oldest treatments known, massage was traditionally a well-recognized part of any treatment regime. It is part of both ayurvedic and Traditional Chinese Medicine and is used by physiotherapists in orthodox medicine. There are also numerous variations of Swedish massage (see below left), the most well known being aromatherapy (see p. 70).

Studies have shown that infants, both animal and human, become physically and psychologically stunted when touch is absent. In a crisis, touch is an automatic part of the support we give others, and is in itself very healing. Massage is quite simply a formalized, focused form of touch.

The therapist will first ask about any particular problems the massage should work on. Also he or she will need to know of infections, inflammations, or current injuries. In pregnancy the stomach and breasts are worked lightly; in cancer the affected area is avoided completely, or worked lightly, since heavy massage can aggravate the condition.

The massage itself will vary with your therapist's training and your needs. It should be neither painfully heavy nor irritatingly light and should not hurt, although there is a pleasurable type of pain that may be felt as the therapist works deeply into tight muscles. Oil, lotion, or talc is used to lubricate the skin. The therapist will feel the tension in your muscles, and this helps determine how much pressure to use. However, feedback is appreciated.

After treatment you may feel sleepy and relaxed, so have some quiet time afterward, to gain full benefit. A good massage affects not only the physical but also the etheric and sometimes the emotional body. Work done at the etheric level has a longer-term effect than a massage that only affects the physical level. The more content you feel after a massage the more the etheric body has been helped.

Massage is a good therapy to try if you enjoy being touched, especially if you are tense. It is also good for the release of muscle tension from sport strains, arthritis, or back problems.

AROMATHERAPY

Aromatherapy is a hands-on therapy combining both massage and the use of essential aromatic oils.

Although sessions include a massage, this is almost secondary to the use of the oils. These have medicinal properties either to improve overall well-being or a specific medical or skin problem. In fact the fragrant essential oils used are not strictly oils, but complex, volatile extracts from plants. They penetrate the skin more completely and have a more profound effect on skin care than oils alone. The aromatic smell also strongly stimulates the limbic, or emotional, centre of the brain, which influences relaxation and the emotions. This part of the brain influences our response to stresses and has a strong effect on psychological and psychosomatic illness. Stimulation from touch, combined with the effects of the oils, can have profound results.

An aromatherapy session usually lasts between one and two hours. Your therapist will first ask about medical problems and any other treatments you are having. Some conditions, such as pregnancy, certain malignancies, and heart disease, are not treated without a doctor's permission. Next the therapist will choose several essential oils according to your complaints, often also including some relaxing or reviving oils. These oils are then mixed into a carrier base. Sometimes you may be asked to smell the oils to aid in the choice, as those you are drawn to are particularly beneficial. Oils are also combined to work over time, some fast-acting and some with a slower but longer-lasting effect.

The massage is usually gentle, with mainly long, sweeping strokes to smooth the oil into the skin. It is better not to have an aromatherapy session straight after exercising since the absorption of the oils will be impeded. Afterward you may feel relaxed and sleepy. Drink plenty of water in the following 24 hours and leave the oils on for several hours for maximum benefit. A course of weekly sessions for a month, and then follow-up sessions as necessary, is often recommended.

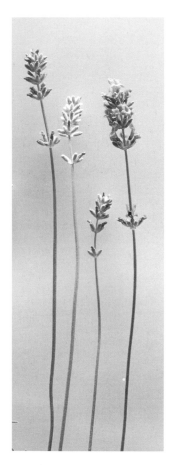

Benefits

Aromatherapy is especially good for psychological conditions such as anxiety and depression, and stress-induced illnesses such as migraines and headaches. It can also help relieve the stress of illness and chronic disease such as cancer.

Skin conditions such as eczema and psoriasis may also respond well to aro-matherapy. The essential oils can also be used for home and first aid treatments, in baths, burners, or inhalations.

OSTEOPATHY

This hands-on treatment uses a range of techniques, including massage, joint mobilization, and manipulation, coupled with advice on posture and lifestyle. Osteopathy theory considers that healing is an innate process that can be supported by treatment, and that all aspects of the human being need to be in balance to generate good health. This is similar to the concept of subtle bodies. Osteopathy treatments are designed to encourage healing to take place at whatever level there is disturbance.

As well as adjustments to joints, osteopaths also use massage and deep pressure to relieve tension, and gentle passive movements to loosen up the body.

Your therapist will ask about current problems, as well as past health, physical problems, accidents, surgery, or injuries and other treatments you may be having. As an osteopath is interested in your whole being you may be asked seemingly unrelated questions; these enable the therapist to determine the origins of your problem.

All osteopaths conduct a physical examination, particularly of your musculoskeletal system, which gives information that cannot be gained by questioning alone. The osteopath works out a course of action, though this may be a referral for further tests, or to another practitioner. Treatment is likely to include light bodywork and then usually the adjustment of joints. The osteopath will ask you to relax and then apply a swift but gentle thrust to restore the normal movement in the joint. To finish you may be given further massage, exercises, and advice to follow at home. This helps strengthen the body and teaches you to avoid situations which may cause recurrences of the problem. Follow-up sessions, intially weekly, may take thirty minutes to one hour. Long-standing conditions often need longer to improve, plus occasional maintenance sessions.

Sometimes there is a healing reaction. This may be a soreness around a manipulation area or a temporary flare-up of your symptoms. If you are concerned you should contact your practitioner.

Theory

Osteopathy was developed by an American doctor, Andrew Taylor Still, in 1894. Disillusioned by the crude and unscientific medicine being practised at that time, he developed osteopathy as an holistic system of healing. It is based on the philosophy that all parts of the body are linked and influenced by all other parts. Also, the structure of the body is linked to its functioning, so if the body structure is out of alignment then the rest of the body cannot function normally.

Benefits

Osteopathy has a well-deserved reputation for backaches and injuries and is good for any problems that involve the musculoskeletal system, such as headache, migraines, and arthritis.

It can also be beneficial for other conditions, especially those with a functional or psychosomatic component such as irritable bowel syndrome, menstrual problems, asthma, and indigestion.

CHIROPRACTIC

This hands-on treatment to adjust displaced joints was developed in the late 1800s in America.

Chiropractic treatment acts on the physical body, which influences the etheric body. Chiropractic theory states that the misalignments of bones, especially the small facet joints protruding from the vertebrae, cause tension in the surrounding tissues. This tension compresses the nerves from the spinal cord that pass close by. These nerves then become irritated, which makes them either more or less electrically active than normal. This change in turn affects the workings of the muscles that the nerves supply, causing pain and stiffness. If the affected nerves supply an organ of the body the electrical changes will upset its normal functioning.

A chiropractic treatment usually consists of a long first session, where symptoms and health problems are discussed. This includes looking at your orthodox doctor's diagnosis, as some conditions are not suitable for chiropractic, including some forms of cancer and arthritis. Particular attention is paid to previous accidents, injuries, or surgery. The chiropractor then examines your posture and the joints of the spine, pelvis, and other major joints. This includes looking at the range of movement, as well as examining the joints. Some chiropractors also take X rays.

The chiropractor will then put you into different positions to expose each joint. The joint is given a sharp tap, directing a physical force into the spine, which allows it to spring back into position. The force used should not be painful; it is often accompanied by a loud click. There may be a temporary flare-up of your symptoms immediately after treatment, but this settles down, usually producing a good long-term result.

Chiropractic is gaining a good reputation for musculoskeletal problems, even in orthodox circles. In addition it is useful in conditions where the symptoms do not obviously relate to the spine, such as migraines, IBS, PMS, and painful menstruation.

McTimoney chiropractic

This is based on similar principles to chiropractic, but uses a slightly different technique to adjust the bones. One hand is placed over the bone to be adjusted and given a glancing strike with the other hand. This method imparts energy to the bone and tissues, which the body can use to reset its skeletal structure. You will hear the noise of the two hands smacking together, but you are unlikely to be aware of the manipulation itself. This technique avoids stretching the ligaments surrounding the bones and minimizes the risk of making the spine less stable and thus more prone to coming out of alignment.

McTimoney practitioners check all the joints at each session, and the therapy is seen as a maintenance practice as much as a treatment.

ROLFING®

Rolfing is a hands-on healing technique that uses deep pressure, applied with the hands or elbows, to particular areas of the body.

In the 1930s Ida Rolf, a biochemist, developed her own philosophy and technique. Originally inspired by yoga, she considered that the organization of the musculoskeletal structure was closely linked to health and wellbeing. Dr Rolf discovered that applying strong pressure over certain areas of the body can release tension, freeing the trapped energy held there that originally caused and still maintains structural distortions. The treatment allows old patterns of holding to be released, whether physical or emotional.

Although devised as a physical technique, Rolfing also affects the etheric and emotional bodies. This may explain how the resolution of old physical problems can activate emotional states.

Treatments are carried out in an exact programme over ten sessions, each one building on the last, enabling the therapist to cover the whole body. The first seven sessions focus on releasing and unravelling distorted structural patterns and each session concentrates on a different part of the body. The last three focus on the reintegration and rebalancing of the musculoskeletal system.

Your therapist will move through a programme, tailored to suit your pattern of tension, checking and treating each part of your body. He or she will modify the approach, depending on what tensions are revealed. As work progresses, you will find that pressure is severe in some areas, where you have resistant holding patterns. Thoughts and feelings may surface, indicating why the tension is there, and your therapist will support you through this release. Afterwards you may feel lighter and freer, both physically and emotionally.

Rolfing was developed as a preventative or maintenance technique, but most clients undertake it because of an illness. The effects are holistic and may deal with other, seemingly unrelated, problems.

Theory

When our skeletal structure is chronically out of alignment we feel stressed, which can result in illness. This misalignment of the bones is often due to unequal tensions held in the myofascia – the system of muscles and connective tissue that holds together the framework of the skeleton and supports the whole body. The aim of Rolfing is to reorganize the myofascia. The technique unravels and rebalances the myofascia tissues.

Benefits

Rolfing is very good for any musculoskeletal problems, especially when emotional states have contributed to the disturbance. It is also effective in treating anxiety states and illnesses which have a psychosomatic component, including migraines, headaches, and asthma. In addition Rolfing helps to minimize the long-term effects of accidents or injuries.

REFLEXOLOGY

In reflexology, thumb pressure on different points of the foot is used to stimulate healing. It is an ancient technique that re-appeared in the 1920s when Dr William Fitzgerald developed a treatment called "zone therapy". This later became known as "reflexology".

According to reflexology theory there is a subtle energy connection, or reflex, between an area of the foot (or hand) and an organ of the body. The soles and tops of the feet and hands are divided into areas representing different parts of the body, shown on a foot map. The idea that part of the body contains a plan for the whole is the ancient idea of the microcosm reflecting the macrocosm.

Reflexology has similarities with acupuncture and shiatsu. Although they are not the same, both "reflexes" and meridians connect the physical to the etheric body. Using pressure on the physical foot releases energy blockages in the etheric body at the true site of the organ as well as on the foot, allowing healing to take place.

Before treatment the therapist will enquire about health problems, noting orthodox diagnosis and treatment. Tell the therapist if you are pregnant – certain areas must be treated with care.

It is extraordinary how much a reflexologist can learn about your health from your feet, and he or she may give you advice about what is discovered. This information is usually recorded on a foot chart. However, reflexology is primarily a treatment, not a diagnostic tool.

Every part of the foot is systematically covered during a treatment. The therapist uses the tip of the thumb in a "crawling" movement to move the point of pressure across the foot. Some areas will be tender and the therapist may feel changes under the skin, indicating problem areas. You should drink plenty of water after the session to help dissipate temporary flare-ups of symptoms. Sometimes a problem will be relieved instantly, but six to eight weekly sessions may be needed for lasting results.

CLASS 2

Apparently physical techniques

reflexology
acupuncture
shiatsu
applied kinesiology

Methods that seem to act directly on the physical body, but in fact access the invisible energy system that interconnects the etheric and physical bodies. They also facilitate changes in the emotional body.

Benefits

Reflexology is especially good for musculoskeletal problems such as backaches, digestive problems, period problems, and problems due to poor lymph drainage. It has also proved useful in treating strokes. Chronic conditions such as arthritis may need regular top-up sessions to maintain a good result.

ACUPUNCTURE

This well-known complementary therapy is part of the 3000-year-old system of Traditional Chinese Medicine, which also includes moxibustion, herbalism, diet, chi kung, and tui na (massage).

In TCM theory life energy (chi) flows along invisible channels of energy known as meridians. Modern research suggests that the meridians lie at the interface between the etheric and physical bodies. It is at this level that Chinese medicine considers disease to arise. In acupuncture fine needles are inserted into the skin at specific points to affect the flow of chi.

You will be asked detailed questions about your symptoms, past problems, and your lifestyle – especially diet and responses to seasons, weather, and time of day. The practitioner will also gain useful information from studying your tongue and pulses at both wrists. Chinese diagnosis can detect energy imbalances in the organ functions before any physical malfunction has taken place. Thus the practitioner can discern which organs are suffering from a deficiency or an excess of chi. Using TCM theory that describes how the internal organs relate to the meridians, the practitioner chooses the points where needles will most effectively free up the energy flow.

Needles are inserted into the chosen points and are usually turned until they produce a sensation known as "deqi", which you may feel as warmth, dullness, tingling, or a sense of expansion. The needles can be left in place from a few minutes to up to half an hour, depending on the treatment. Afterward needle sites may sometimes appear flushed and ooze blood. The acupuncturist views these signs as positive changes in the chi.

Sometimes a smouldering "cigar" of smoking "moxa" (a Chinese herb) is applied to the needles or over an acupuncture point. This is especially used to tonify chi at these points.

An acupuncture session can produce dramatic relief of symptoms, but a course of weekly sessions is usually required to produce and maintain long-term improvement.

Chi flow

Chi flowing freely along the meridians is considered to protect health. Ill health results in a disturbance of this flow. Insertion of needles at points along the meridians has the effect of "tonifying" (stimulating), "sedating" (settling), or "enhancing" (increasing) the chi at these points, which are chosen empirically from many years of traditional practice.

Respect your feelings

Many people find an acupuncture treatment pleasant and relaxing. The needles are quite unlike hypodermic needles, since they are much finer, and puncture rather than cut the skin layer. However some people find the concept of needling threatening. Do respect your body's feelings about this as stress is counterproductive to healing and another method of treatment might be more appropriate.

SHIATSU

Shiatsu, which means "finger pressure", developed in Japan out of 3000-year-old Chinese massage techniques. Traditionally shiatsu has been seen as an aid to maintaining good health rather than a curative therapy and it is used this way today in Japanese medicine. However, it is also valuable as a diagnostic and healing therapy.

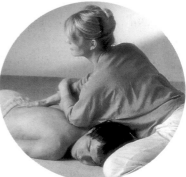

In common with Traditional Chinese Medicine, shiatsu works with the flow of life energy (chi or "ki"), along meridians. At specific points along the meridians the therapist can detect how the ki is disturbed and what treatment is required. Applying pressure to these points moves the ki. Shiatsu works mainly with the etheric via the physical body, but it is also able to influence the higher subtle bodies, as these interact with the etheric body.

Many practitioners start their treatment with little or no information about your health problems and previous treatments. This is because they would rather listen to your body than be confused by your mind. Shiatsu works well with all treatments, even orthodox medicine. There are no contraindications, but treatment of acute injuries and infections may trigger a healing reaction. Sometimes a virus already in your system may become more active after a session. There may appear to be adverse effects, but this is in fact a speeding-up of the healing process.

The therapist begins the treatment kneeling beside you and moves around you as the treatment progresses. The therapist's movements are an important part of the treatment. The use of his or her body weight, breathing pattern, and personal energy, or Ki, is as necessary as the use of the hands.

During the treatment you are encouraged to close your eyes and absorb all physical sensations. The treatment not only involves applying pressure to the body but also moving the head and limbs in order to maximize the effects of the pressure.

The treatment is very relaxing. Afterward your body often feels freer and looser and you have a sense of serenity, wholeness, and wellbeing.

Benefits

Shiatsu can be helpful in any condition, but is particularly beneficial for migraines, anxiety attacks, breathing problems, digestive problems, insomnia, and general aches and pains.

Shiatsu's main strength is that it can complement other treatments. This is because it concentrates on strengthening healthiness rather than attacking the disease. Also it can often help you unravel what is wrong with your health rather than just treating symptoms.

APPLIED KINESIOLOGY

Muscle strengthening

A variety of techniques is used to strengthen the muscles, which in itself restores energy balance. These include deep massage to affect lymph drainage from the muscle, light touch on neurovascular points or acupuncture points, or gentle sweeping over a meridian.

After each technique the muscle is retested. If a muscle is particularly difficult to strengthen you may be given exercises, or lifestyle changes may be suggested.

Applied kinesiology (AK) is an apparently physical technique that uses muscle strength to test for energy imbalances and localized massage or touch to correct this balance. The technique was developed by an American chiropractor, Dr George Goodheart, in 1964.

Muscle strength is a good indicator of wellbeing as the tone or resting tension of a muscle is directly linked to the mind and emotions and our internal chemistry. Dr Goodheart discovered that testing the strength of different muscles could detect problems that did not seem to affect them directly. It became apparent that this system was tapping into the energy flow in the body in much the same way as Traditional Chinese Medicine treats chi flow in the meridians. The strength of the muscles tested seems to relate to the free flow of energy through the meridian that passes over that muscle.

An AK session lasts up to an hour. Muscles are tested one at a time: the practitioner will ask you to hold your arm or leg in the position that exercises the muscle. He or she will then gently press or pull on the limb while you resist. If you are unable to hold the position this indicates a disturbance to the energy flow through the muscle.

To begin with the practitioner will use an arm muscle to check that your body is responding accurately. He or she will then test at least fourteen muscles, each relating to a different acupuncture meridian and internal organ. These tests indicate which muscles need strengthening to bring your body into energetic balance. The session is complete when the muscles tested are all at normal strength.

Food allergies and nutritional deficiencies are sometimes the cause of persistent weakness. You may be asked to hold a food or supplement while the muscle is retested, which may indicate that a food exclusion or a supplement may be necessary.

Chronic emotional states can also cause persistent muscle weakness and your practitioner may practise various emotional stress release techniques.

REIKI

Reiki is a hands-on healing method developed in Japan at the beginning of the twentieth century by scholar and theologian, Mikao Usui. He suggested a set prescription for using the hands, while energy is used by the client's deeper levels of consciousness for whatever it is most needed – physical, emotional, or spiritual health. The ability to practise reiki is not taught, but is an empowering by a Master. This is an energy transfer given through touch, in four "initiations", which open up energy centres in the body so that the channelling of the reiki energy becomes easy and safe. This energy is usually felt in the hands as heat, vibration, or tingling.

Reiki energy appears to be the same as prana or chi and is freely used by the receiver to aid healing in any or all of the subtle bodies, although the giver does not decide what needs to be "fixed". He or she may ask you about orthodox treatments, but the reiki itself will provide feedback about what is wrong. The giver may use light massage, but mainly places the hands over parts of the body, usually beginning at the head. The hands are held for a few minutes on each position and you may feel warmth, coldness, or tingling. Normally the whole body is covered, starting on the front, in a session lasting between half and one hour. You may fall asleep; occasionally tears are shed, but these are more of a release than an exposure of emotional problems. Afterward you may feel relaxed or energized.

Reiki can be done daily, but frequency of sessions will be influenced by time and money. More experienced therapists can channel reiki at a distance. For chronic complaints weekly sessions are very effective, allowing for healing to continue and for healing reactions such as headaches, nausea, or diarrhoea to clear. Chronic conditions may take time to improve, but the effects of accidents and acute illnesses may clear up in only one session. Healing may not necessarily be on a physical level. In terminal illness reiki can be valuable to help the person come to a peaceful resolution to life.

CLASS 3
Light touch techniques

reiki
spiritual healing
therapeutic touch

Methods that barely, if at all, touch the physical body and that aim to influence the etheric body directly. They also make it easier for you to make changes in your emotional and mental bodies and for you to contact your causal body.

Benefits

Reiki can be used for any illnesses or injuries, as well as emotional upsets and spiritual confusion. The receiver uses the energy wherever it is most needed.

Reiki works well with other therapies, including orthodox medicine. It is very good as a self-help tool and you can give it to yourself or to your family and friends. Reiki training courses at different levels are held throughout the world. For personal use the First Degree course is sufficient.

SPIRITUAL HEALING

Benefits

Spiritual healing can be an excellent way of relieving stress, a precursor for much illness, especially psycho-somatic and psychological diseases such as headaches, migraines, IBS, asthma, anxiety, and depression. It is used widely to help relieve emotional pain such as bereavement. It can also be of value in difficult-to-treat conditions such as cancer, chronic fatigue syndrome, and multiple sclerosis.

Spiritual healing is a form of light-touch healing. In its present form, it has become an umbrella term for a number of light-touch healing techniques claiming to work by channelling the healing energy of the cosmos through the healer, for the benefit of those being healed. This may be through the hands, or at a distance by visualization and prayer.

Spiritual healing can be done either individually or in a group session. A one-to-one session usually lasts around 30 minutes. The healer places his or her hands on your shoulders to tune in to your causal body, which starts the energy flow through the healer's hands. The energy is directed to six of the chakras, from the brow downward, by holding the hands a little way from the body over each chakra area in turn. This brings the chakras into balance, activating the natural healing mechanisms.

As well as holding feelings of compassion and the focus of intent to heal, your healer will experience the sensation of the energy flow through your body. During the healing you may also feel these sensations. The most usual are tingling, warmth, and coolness. Finally, the healing is concluded by the healer's hands returning to your shoulders. After the healing you should drink a glass of water, which helps the physical body discharge any toxins released by the healing.

Some healers combine other healing techniques with the basic spiritual healing. These sessions are usually an hour long and allow for more time to be spent listening to your problems, on the healing itself, and dealing with anything that may have come up emotionally during the session. Sessions at two-week intervals are usual, to allow assimilation.

Between sessions your healer may ask you to practise meditation, relaxation, or visualization exercises to help you learn simply to "be". This is the state where self-healing can best take place. For many, experience with this type of healing opens up their own desires to heal others. This may be an undeveloped gift from childhood which reveals itself.

THERAPEUTIC TOUCH

Therapeutic touch (TT) uses the hands to direct life energy to the patient in order to encourage natural healing. A reworking of the ancient practice of the laying-on of hands, it was developed in the USA in the 1970s by Dora Kunz and Dr Dolores Krieger.

TT is based on the widely held energy-healing theory that we all exist in a "sea" of life energy, which constantly supplies us with the energy we call "life". This same theory also considers that we are more than just our physical body. TT is a means of directing the body's subtle life energy back into balance. The effect of this on the physical level is the restoration of wellbeing and health.

TT practitioners are trained to use their energy field as a conduit between the sea of life energy and the patient's energy field. They tap into the life energy and simply direct it to areas that need it, where it is used to balance, unblock, or restore deficiencies in the receiver's energy field. This boosts the body's natural healing and the effect filters through to the consciousness as relief or cure of physical symptoms or mental distress.

The therapist will work with what they find in your energy field. After gently massaging your shoulders to help you relax, he or she will make a slow, sweeping motion, head to feet, with the hands a short distance from the body. This "reads" your energy field and also marks the beginning of the rebalancing process. Next the hands move to areas where energy disturbance has been noticed – not necessarily corresponding to painful or diseased areas. Your therapist may again touch you and ask you to visualize a colour or scene.

Finally your overall field is rechecked. During the treatment you may notice breathing changes, a feeling of expansion or heaviness, muscles twitching, a rumbling stomach, plus heat or tingling, the arousal of emotions, or mental images – all signs that changes are taking place in your subtle bodies. After the treatment most people experience a sense of peace and wellbeing.

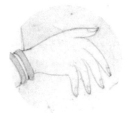

Benefits

Therapeutic touch is used in hospital intensive care units since it is very good for helping wounds, infections, and injuries to heal faster. It is also good for headaches, psychosomatic and stress-related symptoms, and is an excellent treatment for emotional distress. An invaluable treatment for the terminally ill, it helps in pain relief and overcoming the fear of dying.

Acute conditions respond well to treatment, which is best given daily. The very ill benefit from short, frequent treatments. Chronic conditions need weekly treatments, though it may take several weeks before the effects are noticeable.

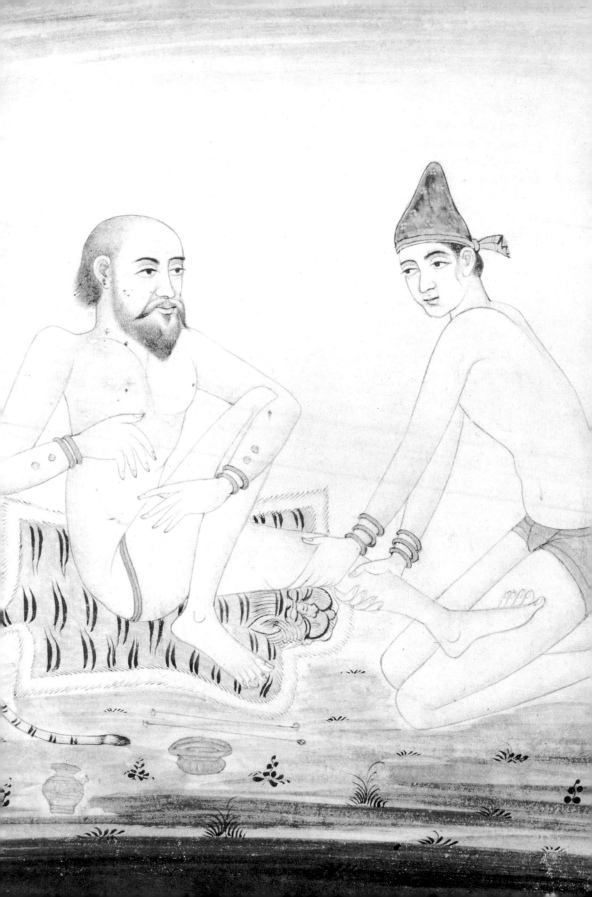

YOGA

The word "yoga" is Sanskrit for "yoke", or "union". Yoga is an aspect of ayurveda originating in India 4000 years ago and designed to bring union between mind, body, and spirit. Of the many schools of yoga, probably the most well known is hatha yoga. All types of yoga aim to achieve the bliss of being at one with everything (samadi).

The postures (asanas) of hatha yoga are excellent for developing and maintaining flexibility and muscle strength. They are also a good way to relax. At this physical level yoga contributes a great deal to fitness and wellbeing. However yoga asanas are designed not just to work on the physical body but also on the subtle bodies. Because there is a focus on inner awareness of breathing and the internal sensations, as well as the physical positions themselves, this activates the etheric body more strongly than ordinary exercise. The activation also extends into the emotional and mental bodies. The aim of the asanas is to align these bodies, helping to restore health wherever in the subtle bodies the originating problem might be. Yoga can also be used to increase connection with your causal body.

Even if you have a specific illness, a yoga class is a good way to improve health, as most of the common poses are useful to everyone. However there are some conditions, such as high blood pressure, pregnancy, menstruation, and back problems that certain postures do not suit. Most classes start with standing postures, for warming up and developing strength, and then move on to sitting postures. Postures are normally done slowly and held for a while. They should not be forced to the point of pain, but should extend you.

Beginners' classes finish with a relaxation pose, while more advanced classes move on to pranayama (see p. 92) and meditation (see p. 109). Classes are usually one and a half to two hours long and for real progress weekly classes are necessary. It is also very beneficial to do a few minutes' practice daily as well – your teacher may suggest suitable postures.

CLASS 4
Active methods/disciplines

yoga
Alexander technique
tai chi
chi kung

Methods involving a physical discipline that you learn and practise. These techniques set down an ideal for your body to attain, whatever it is capable of at present. Though apparently physical, these techniques affect all the energy bodies. The focus is on first making changes in the etheric body.

Benefits

The asanas of hatha yoga can help to prevent and treat degenerative diseases, especially arthritis and osteoporosis. They are also good for treating psychosomatic illnesses such as asthma, migraine, eczema, and irritable bowel syndrome. The asanas are also effective for anxiety, depression, and addictions, and as a self-help discipline to relieve and deal with stress.

Any illness may be improved by yoga as it aids physical, emotional, and mental wellbeing. This will occur whether or not you are practising pranayama or meditation as well.

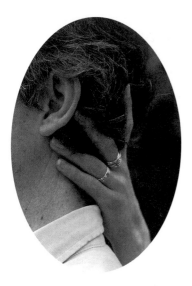

ALEXANDER TECHNIQUE

Alexander technique (AT) is a light-touch technique developed in the 1930s by Frederick Alexander. Its practitioners see it as a process of re-education in the use of the body.

Most of us think that our movement is dependent on muscles contracting – by developing tension. AT trains you to make this type of simple movement without this happening, by first changing your position so that your joints are in balance. When a joint is held in balance the muscles either side of the joint work in synchrony, so as one relaxes the other contracts effortlessly.

Alexander technique may appear physical, but it mainly works on the etheric and the mental body. The teacher's hands gently guide the movements of the physical body, in the process freeing up any distorting influences from the emotional body that are creating tension in the physical body.

The technique is a tool for you to develop to help yourself. A "lesson" begins with minimal discussion of problems. Your teacher will then guide you through a series of repeated movements, watching how you use your body and how this distorts your posture. You soon become familiar with the sequence that the teacher's hands are guiding you through. Your role is not passive, though you may notice joints and muscles shifting unexpectedly under this gentle guidance. As you move, you will be asked to be consciously aware of three suggestions. These are that the neck be free, the head moves forward and upward, and the back lengthens and widens. When you keep these in mind at the same time as you perform the body movements, the two become linked in your subconscious and inefficient patterns of movement are replaced.

The lessons are usually half an hour weekly. You are encouraged to be aware of the mental suggestions as you go about your daily life between lessons. A course of 30 to 40 lessons will give you enough of a base to continue on your own, but fewer sessions can still be beneficial.

Benefits

AT is very good for sufferers of chronic back problems and arthritis. It also helps headaches, migraines, and some visual problems – all aggravated by tension in the back of the neck, which Alexander technique is particularly able to relieve. Its role in correcting postural problems, especially when awkward positions have to be maintained for long periods, makes it popular with dancers and musicians.

TAI CHI

Tai chi chuan originated in China as a martial art and the name roughly translates as "cosmic fist", referring to the fact that the technique derives its power from the energy of the Universe. In China it is considered the most advanced form of the martial arts and is still widely practised today as a health maintenance technique.

Tai chi is a body movement technique that uses the physical body and mind to affect the energy of the whole of your being (chi). The practice makes you increasingly aware of the etheric body and gives you the ability to both feel and control the chi as it moves at this level. Tai chi also brings the emotional body into alignment with the rest of the subtle bodies, particularly via the mental body.

In the West there has been a tendency to concentrate on the health aspect (yin) rather than the martial art aspect (yang). Unless both aspects are developed in balance the technique loses most of its ability to enhance health, though wellbeing can be achieved. Therefore a good teacher is essential.

There are five aspects to tai chi training, although many teachers only practise some of them. The most familiar is known as the "form" (tao chuan). This is a fluid series of movements, each having a name that describes its purpose and shape. This series is learned and performed with attention not only to its external shape and movement sequence but also to the inner experience of weight shift, co-ordination of breathing, and visualization.

Although tai chi practice builds over the years, a year of practice should show considerable benefits. With time a very real experience of the movement of chi energy is perceived, together with the ability to direct and control the interaction between yin and yang in the body, which is what produces the movement of chi. It is this ability that gives tai chi its strength as a martial art.

Other aspects of tai chi are "pushing hands" (tui shou), self defence (san shou), weapons training, and internal strength exercises (nei kung).

Benefits

Tai chi is particularly good for protecting and relieving degenerative, psychosomatic, and psychiatric illness. Conditions such as asthma, arthritis, gastritis, rheumatism, migraines, depression, and nervousness can all be helped by tai chi. It is very much a self-help technique, so it needs the discipline of committed practice.

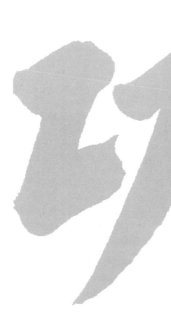

CHI KUNG

Benefits

The beneficial effects from regular practice of chi kung can be noticed after just a few weeks and within two or three months significant improvement should be apparent. There is the almost immediate benefit of relaxation when stressed and revitalization when tired. Over longer periods it can help arthritis, anxiety, and depression, chronic fatigue syndrome, and psychosomatic illnesses such as headaches or irritable bowel syndrome.

Chi kung also supports any other therapy, particularly other aspects of TCM such as acupuncture (see p. 75) or Chinese herbalism (see p. 117).

Chi kung is based on the Traditional Chinese Medicine theory of yin and yang, chi flow, and meridians (see pp. 42–6). It is designed to stimulate the flow of chi (energy) through the body by synchronizing simple movements with breathing. The origins of chi kung are lost in time, but it seems to be more ancient than tai chi. Its movements were developed as a self-healing, or health maintenance, system, while tai chi originated as a martial art.

The movements and breathing of chi kung encourage maximum movement of chi through the cycle of yang and yin, as well as the free flow of chi along the meridians. This energizes the body as a whole and also stimulates the functioning of each organ. The effect is probably generated at the level of the physical and etheric bodies, but the changes here also influence the outer subtle bodies, which accounts for its calming and meditative effects.

Classes begin with simple, repetitive warm-up exercises to relax your body, especially the waist area, where chi is "stored". This area is called "tan tien" and your breathing is focused here.

The moves have some similarity to those of tai chi. The main difference is that the feet are rarely moved in chi kung. The core exercises are a series of slow movements co-ordinated with breathing. Each one focuses on one particular aspect of the flow of chi, for example along a specific meridian, with benefits for individual organs. You may learn a set of general vitalizing or relaxing exercises, or exercises that benefit a particular health problem.

Once you have mastered some routines it is good to incorporate them into your daily life. Ten to fifteen minutes' daily practice is sufficient to produce significant benefit and making a regular time for exercise is ideal – first thing in the morning is a good time. However the simplicity of the exercises makes them suitable to do at work if you have a few minutes of quiet time. This can boost your energy, and at the same time be relaxing when you are in the middle of a stressful task.

FIVE RHYTHMS DANCE™

This dance technique was developed by Gabrielle Roth in the 1970s. Technically it is a modern dance method, with no direct relation to healing, but it can also be a powerful tool for self-healing.

The theory is that all movement can be separated out into five styles, composing a cycle moving from stillness through movement and back to stillness again. Each of the movements is associated with different emotions and sensations. "Flowing" (strong, fluid, sinuous) has a powerful, almost erotic, energy, generating fear or excitement, while "staccato" (abrupt, direct) has a more aggressive, masculine feel, encouraging the development of boundaries and which can generate anger. "Chaos" (fixed foot patterns while the body is released into chaotic frenzy) is a place of hell, ecstasy, and change, while "lyrical" (flowing, but based on a skipping foot pattern) is joy, release, lightness. Finally, "stillness" (slow movements slowing into stillness, or faster movements resolving into a still space) is peace, calm, meditation, or sometimes, inertia. Each theme can be developed endlessly.

By working with these movements, to appropriate music, it is possible to express the body's physical range of movements and also the full range of emotions and sensations. This allows exploration and release of denied or trapped feelings. For some this physical approach is a far more effective way of accessing feelings than mind-orientated techniques. The technique also generates inner balance more usually achieved by meditation. This state is called "moving stillness" and is a centring within the physical, etheric, emotional, and mental bodies, allowing for deeper connection to the causal body.

Sessions are often in quite large groups, which adds to the power of the experience. Five rhythms dance cannot be fully considered a "therapy" as little guidance or support is given. In this respect it is much closer to a shamanic training. The dance creates altered states of consciousness in which healing, particularly emotional healing, can occur.

CLASS 5
Active methods/dance

five rhythms dance™
trance dance
eurythmy

Methods that involve free physical movement, which increases the movement of energy in the body, in turn enhancing our emotional experience. These therapies give access to the emotional body and provide an opportunity to release or express buried feelings and experience changes in consciousness affecting the mental bodies.

Benefits

Five rhythms dance can be used to support more active healing methods such as orthodox medicine, homeopathy, or psychotherapy. It is useful for psychological illness, especially depression, but then it should be backed up with a one-to-one treatment such as psychotherapy. Psychosomatic and chronic illness, such as migraines, irritable bowel syndrome, chronic fatigue syndrome, and asthma, may also benefit.

Benefits

Although trance dance does not claim to cure illness it can help other, more treatment-orientated, methods to work, as it frees up the connection to the causal body and the healing energies that lie beyond. It is particularly useful as an adjunct to psychological therapies as it provides a balance for these mind-orientated approaches. Trance dance is not suitable for people suffering from serious mental illness and does require a basic level of physical health sufficient to make dancing possible.

TRANCE DANCE

Trance dance is the new name given to an old form of dancing originating from the merging of West African dance and music traditions with the Sufi tradition in Morocco, and with Brazilian traditions. In the 1980s the tradition was brought into the field of psychology and healing by Dr David Akstein.

The dance can continue for hours and alter states of consciousness, using a specific rhythm (cross-rhythm), which is too complex for the logical brain to analyze. This distracts the dominant left brain and enables the right and left hemispheres to harmonize. Such harmonization opens up the opportunity for a profound change in consciousness, enabling connection with our causal bodies and beyond that to cosmic consciousness, or the "divine". In this transcendent state profound healing can occur on mental, emotional, or physical levels. Thus trance dance can affect any of the subtle bodies. The effect is directed subconsciously to where it is needed.

Trance dance is a group experience and usually takes place in a series of sessions. The music is a unique blend of its original roots and incorporates drumming and singing. Participants form groups of four or five and one person from the group dances in each session. The non-dancing members support and protect the dancer, so that he or she can dance freely, with eyes closed. The dancer is "induced" into the dance by gently rotating the upper body and then being spun round to assist induction into an altered state of consciousness. He or she is then encouraged to dance freely and spontaneously. Once this happens there is a change in consciousness.

Initially emotions trapped in the emotional body may arise and be experienced intensely, but as the dance moves on, and over repeated sessions, these give way to higher or transcendental experiences such as love and joy, laughter, bliss, and a different perspective on life. The process continues for long afterward. It is an excellent method of moving your spiritual unfoldment to another level, particularly if it has become stuck.

EURYTHMY

This movement therapy is based on anthroposophy, (see p. 97) developed by Rudolf Steiner.

A therapist can recognize "disease pattern" by the way you move, and can tailor a "treatment pattern" of movements to restore your instinctive way of moving. Movement has a strong effect on the flow of energy at the etheric level, especially when attention is focused at this level. The change in energy flow affects the higher subtle bodies and corrects the activities of the body, because the physical body mimics the energy pattern of the etheric body.

Eurythmy is taught in groups and individual sessions. The fundamental use of sound is as single syllables which carry the essence of the pure form of the movements. The therapist will make the sound, but the clients practise in silence, visualizing the sound and appropriate associations to it as they carry out the movement. Eurythmy movements are fluid, but they can be vigorous and include jumps.

Group sessions usually focus on stress release and revitalization movements rather than individual treatments. The group works together or in couples and may use props such as balls or copper rods. The effect is that of a moving group meditation, bringing relaxation, revitalization, and insight.

Individual sessions are a chance to tailor a movement programme specific to your health requirements. Initially the teacher asks about past and present medical problems, treatments, and your life. You may be asked to perform simple eurythmy exercises. This will help the teacher decide what movements will be most appropriate and you will learn a sequence of these at subsequent sessions. You need to learn both the physical aspect of the movement and also its inner feel, practising at home between sessions. It usually takes between five and ten sessions to grasp the whole sequence. You then practise at home for ten to twelve weeks before taking a two- or three-week break to allow the process to deepen subconsciously. The sequence is then restarted.

Benefits

Eurythmy can be used to treat all manner of illnesses. Asthma and respiratory problems, and arthritis are particularly quick to respond. While the disease may not be eliminated, eurythmy is very good at minimizing flare-ups. Other diseases for which it is widely used are strokes, high blood pressure, cancer, and depression. It has been found to be especially helpful in the treatment of chronic fatigue syndrome and also in preparation for surgery, with the effect of speeding post-operative recovery.

Methods that involve the
therapist moving the
body, which can affect
the overall energy flow in
the etheric and emotional
bodies.

FELDENKRAIS METHOD

In Feldenkrais students perform exercises designed to focus attention on "how" they move. Normally instructions are given verbally, though sometimes the teacher will also use touch to guide the student to a deeper realization of how they are moving.

The method was developed by the physicist and judo teacher, Moshe Feldenkrais, in the 1940s. He believed that thinking, perception, and emotion are inextricably linked to our actions and that the easiest way to learn about the Self was by observing our habitual ways of doing things. He also believed that it is easiest to change our way of being through changing our actions. Knowing oneself is an ancient tool for spiritual growth and Feldenkrais's work taps into this concept. In this way it links in with the theories of body energy fields or subtle bodies.

Feldenkrais lessons can be taken individually or in groups. The efficient way of moving that the lessons encourage is not taught as a formula but is explored by each individual. Students are encouraged to become aware of their own habitual actions and to discover new possibilities. The actions are done repetitively or in incremental stages, to enhance perception of the sensations of what happens in every part of the body. In this way the student can build up a more extensive awareness of what happens during an action, allowing for new choices in how to function. The awareness not only affects posture and movements but also gives poise and wellbeing to the emotions, perceptions, and thinking. This creates an opening of consciousness that can be a door to healing.

Individual lessons are structured in the same way, although there is more opportunity for the teacher to focus on the student's unique needs, using touch as well as voice. Lessons are usually about 45 minutes each week. Since people respond individually to the Feldenkrais method, the number of lessons needed varies. Usually students continue until they find a place of improvement that feels right. They may come back later for additional learning.

Benefits

Feldenkrais appeals to a wide range of people. Some, such as those in the performing arts, use the method to improve their ability. It is also very beneficial for generalized aches and stiffness such as back problems, arthritis, or old injuries. Sufferers from anxiety, stress, and illnesses with a significant psycho-somatic component may find the method beneficial. It can also help serious neurological problems such as cerebral palsy, multiple sclerosis, or neuromuscular disorders.

BIODYNAMIC MASSAGE

This healing technique combines psychotherapy with hands-on physical methods of massage. Its founder, Gerda Boysen, was originally a psychotherapist, but was inspired by Reichian treatment to develop bio-dynamic massage.

A biodynamic therapist receives training both in psychotherapy and hands-on body techniques, including different types of massage, deep pressure point work, holding and passive movements of the head or limbs. Sometimes more subtle energy work is done by simply placing the hands on different parts of the body.

Sessions last an hour and in the first the therapist usually sets up a "contract" for a fixed number of sessions, after which treatment is reviewed. The chief purpose of the initial session is to ascertain what you wish to achieve.

The therapist will note your body posture, your unconscious movements – especially breathing patterns – and how your body reacts to what you talk about. Once massage begins, subtle indicators such as the tone, texture, and colour of skin, and areas of heat or coldness are also noted. This allows the therapist to make an intuitive decision on which areas and which techniques will help you release trapped energy, which is contributing to your symptoms.

You will be encouraged to talk about what you are experiencing and your therapist may guide you deeper into that experience. You may notice physical release during the treatment such as changes in bowel sounds and breathing patterns. Some more dramatic changes might be relief of physical pain, involuntary muscle movements, shaking, or deep emotions manifesting as tears, laughter, or rage.

This therapy is not confrontational, but supports you in your process of releasing trapped energies. As time goes on the emphasis of the sessions may become more psychological than physical, but all the methods are aimed at re-establishing the free flow of energy through the etheric body, which is essential for good health.

Theory

Biodynamic massage is based on the idea that in illness life energy becomes trapped in the bones, connective tissue, and muscles. This pattern on the physical level reflects energy held in the etheric body. Such energy distortion is often set up by emotional habit patterns or unresolved emotional issues.

The energy released during biodynamic massage also releases the trapped energy back into the emotional body. This makes your conscious mind aware of these emotional patterns, so that they can be expressed freely and seen for what they are.

Benefits

Biodynamic massage is particularly helpful for functional or psychosomatic disorders such as IBS, asthma, headaches, migraines, digestive problems, arthritis, and back problems. It is particularly appropriate when the illness is directly affecting the posture or use of the body, for example with asthma.

ZERO BALANCING

Zero balancing (ZB) is a hands-on healing technique which uses pressure on the body or held stretches of the limbs to affect the energy body and so influence health and wellbeing. It was developed in the 1970s by Fritz Smith MD, who had trained in a wide range of complementary therapies. From this experience he developed his own technique, loosely described as structural acupressure, or ZB.

ZB recognizes that the physical body is associated with an energy body whose integrity is essential for physical wellbeing. Although this energy system is not based on the four layers of subtle bodies, it does recognize that the mind and emotions, as well as physical structure, affect health and wellbeing. The techniques of ZB are designed to interact with the energy body at the level that is appropriate for healing. This may be physical, or at a mental or emotional level. The aim is to restore the equilibrium recognized physically as "health".

A ZB session will begin with the therapist asking about your illness and other treatments. Initially your back and sacroiliac joints will be examined for imbalances. The technique uses gentle pressure to the body or gentle held traction to the limbs, known as "essential touch". This and a "fulcrum" balancing technique is used to evaluate the load-bearing joints where there is little movement (such as the sacroiliac joint) and then to rebalance them, before checking to evaluate the response.

Your therapist will watch for physical signs that indicate that your energy bodies are responding. The tension in your joints, eye movements, breathing, and other physical signs such as a rumbling stomach all indicate a rebalancing of your energy. The practitioner will also sense changes directly through his or her hands. By the end of the session you should feel serene and contented.

ZB sessions are usually around half an hour long, depending on your structural and energetic needs. It is recommended that you start with weekly sessions for four weeks and then review your needs.

Benefits

ZB is particularly useful as a health-maintenance system since it promotes relaxation and stress relief and also reintegrates the physical and energy bodies.

An effective treatment for back or joint problems, it is also helpful for psycho-somatic illnesses such as migraines, asthma, and irritable bowel syndrome. It is very good for psychological problems such as anxiety or depression, or simply to help us handle mentally or emotionally difficult times.

ZB can produce as profound emotional or mental changes as psychotherapy, although the treatment is entirely body-orientated. This makes it suitable for people who do not wish to delve into their psyche to deal with psychological difficulties.

PRANAYAMA

Pranayama is not a therapy in the usual sense, though practitioners can gain great health benefits. The simple translation of pranayama is "breath control". It is an aspect of hatha yoga (see p. 82), following on from the postures, or asanas. It is not a beginner's practice and must not be taken lightly.

Prana translates from the Sanskrit as "life's breath", but it means more. It is also a description of the life force of the Universe energizing animate and inanimate objects. So pranayama is not just a breathing exercise, but more a way of moving and distributing life force around the body, along a network of energy channels called the "nadis".

Patterns of pranayama increase the flow of prana into the physical and subtle bodies and also balance the flow within these. This produces physiological changes in the physical body and also psychological effects, for example improving memory and creativity. These changes can both maintain and improve health.

Pranayama should be done in a sitting position, spine upright. There are several yoga postures that allow this, but the ideal is the full lotus, though the half lotus is perfectly acceptable. The eyes are closed and the mind is focused on the inner experience. In many of the exercises the fingers and thumbs are used to close the nostrils gently, while in some they form special hand positions known as "mudras". Another technique used is to tighten muscles around a body orifice such as the throat. This is a "bandha", which enhances the effectiveness of breathing.

It is inappropriate to use pranayama without the foundation of the yoga asanas as these are a preparation for this more advanced practice. For this reason pranayama is normally taught in advanced yoga classes in addition to the asanas and not on its own. Pranayama can be used to enhance the ability to control the mind or the ego. This then helps the practitioner move on to the more subtle yoga practices, the concentration (dharana), meditation (dhyana), and state of bliss (samadi).

CLASS 7
Breathing techniques

pranayama
rebirthing

Methods that use breathing patterns to enhance and change the energy flow in the body. These methods have the potential to access all the energy bodies.

Benefits
Pranayama is a way of boosting the improvement to health that yoga asanas provide. It is especially useful for psychosomatic illnesses, particularly digestive problems. It is also very helpful for respiratory problems such as asthma and its effect on overall health and wellbeing complements other therapies.

REBIRTHING

Rebirthing is a way of using the breath to access states of consciousness normally unavailable to us. This allows trapped patterns of energy, which can contribute to psychological difficulties or illness, to be released. It was first developed in the 1970s by Leonard Orr.

The process of rebirthing is not theoretically based on the subtle bodies, but can be viewed as accessing every part of this energy system, especially the etheric and emotional bodies. Once it has cleared trapped energy in the lower bodies, it is common for the effects to move to the mental body, so that thought can be observed in a similar way to meditation. It is also a powerful tool to access the causal body.

The initial session includes a questionnaire on goals, health and mental state, and any drug use. Rebirthing must not be practised under the influence of alcohol or social drugs. Heart disease, severe lung problems, and mental illness are also contraindications. Follow-up sessions are mainly devoted to the breathwork. Your practitioner will endeavour to provide whatever you need, so that you can let go of normal waking consciousness.

The experiences of a rebirthing session are diverse, but generally it is initially hard work to keep up with the breathing cycles. Feelings of discomfort, tingling, numbness, and coldness are common and you are encouraged to breath through these sensations. As they pass, warmth and relaxation often follow and the breathing starts to become easier. Many people then enter an emotional phase, where trapped emotions, often grief, come to the fore. Your breathing needs to be kept in focus and your practitioner will help you with this and to relax into the emotion until it passes. Next you may reach a calm or meditative state, or even sleep. Here thoughts can be calmly observed and bliss-type states can occur. Once the process has been completed your practitioner will gently talk you back into normal consciousness.

Theory

A truly healthy in-and-out breath is a smooth process. Emotional traumas in the past may have caused us to hold our breath at the time, and this pattern sticks at a subliminal level in our breathing pattern.

If you concentrate on your breathing, taking the in-and-out breath a little further than normal and repeating the cycle, the stuck patterns begin to show up and the energy trapped in them is released.

Benefits

Rebirthing is a useful tool for personal growth and in treating stress-related illness such as psychosomatic illnesses and psychological problems. It is also very helpful in dealing with stressful illness, such as terminal and chronic disease, and has been used to treat chronic fatigue syndrome.

HOMEOPATHY

Homeopathy is a well-established complementary therapy, though some homeopaths are orthodox doctors, too. It originated in the early 1800s with an orthodox German doctor, Samuel Hahnemann, who derived his remedies mainly from herbs and also mineral and animal products. Homeopathy grew out of Hahnemann's ideas on illness and healing. He believed that illness was due to a disturbance in the life force of the body, and that his prepared remedies neutralized this disturbance. The remedies were developed from three concepts. The first was that "like cures like". This is an ancient concept, but Hahnemann looked at it again after noticing that if he took quinine, a known treatment for malaria, he experienced malaria symptoms.

The second concept was that small doses are more effective than large doses. In Hahnemann's time problems with side effects from herbal mixtures were common and this was an attempt to minimize them. The highly dilute preparations statistically do not contain a single molecule of the original substance. This is why there is no danger of poisoning, even when very poisonous substances, such as arsenic, are used. However, in recent years it has been confirmed that the preparations do have measurable physical effects on living organisms. It has been suggested that this effect is caused by a patterning in the water caused by "succussion" (see p. 95), which is a unique part of the process of making homeopathic remedies of different potencies.

Homeopathic remedies are made from the starter substance by either making a strong solution of the substance or, if it is insoluble, grinding it very finely. If in solution it is then diluted either 1 in 10 (which ultimately makes an "X" or a "D" dilution remedy) or 1 in 100 parts (which makes a "C" dilution remedy). The finely ground insoluble substances are ground with "sac lac" (milk sugar) in the same ratios 100 times. This is known as "trituration". After three triturations the mix is dissolved in water and treated as a soluble substance.

CLASS 8
Water programming

homeopathy
Bach flower remedies
anthroposophy

Methods that act on the subtle bodies by direct communication with them, using energy patterns held in water.

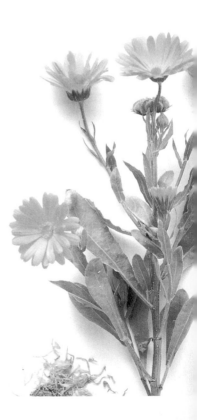

Benefits

Homeopathy is traditionally used for any type of chronic, long-term illness. It seems particularly effective in certain people, especially children. Homeopathy is also important in the treatment of acute and everyday ailments such as injuries, colds, stomach upsets, coughs, and any sort of viral illness. These are conditions that orthodox medicine has little to offer in the way of treatment.

Next the mixture is shaken vigorously, usually by banging it on a hard surface, 100 times – the process known as "succussion". The number of times this process of diluting takes place is the number placed in front of the X, D, or C on the remedy bottle, and is referred to as the "potency" of the remedy. Not all dilutions are used, as it was found that in practice some were more effective than others. Sometimes potencies higher than 200C are used. These are the M, or 1-in-1000 dilution, or even CM (1-in-100,000) potencies. These remedies are made using a machine, as the traditional way would take too long.

It is generally considered that higher potencies (greater dilutions) of remedies have their primary effect on the emotional, and possibly mental, bodies while the lower potencies affect the etheric body, but in practice many homeopaths tend to use what works best for them.

A homeopathy consultation involves questions about your ailments, your approach to life, your illness and personal preferences, especially about foods, weather, times of the day and year, and also detailed questions about past health, life events, and lifestyle. From this information the practitioner can match up you and your condition to the remedy whose "symptom picture" fits best. Every homeopathic remedy has a symptom picture that has been collected by observation and recorded in various homeopathic Materia Medica.

Follow-up is usually done monthly, when the medication is reviewed. The remedies are often changed during the course of treatment as different aspects of the illness come to light. The treatment is usually given as tablets, powders to be dissolved in the mouth, or occasionally, as drops. These need to be handled, stored, and taken carefully, as they are entirely composed of subtle energy patterns and these are easily disrupted. The course of medicines may be as short as a single dose, though it is more common for them to be taken longer-term on a daily or weekly basis.

BACH FLOWER REMEDIES

The Bach flower remedies comprise 38 preparations made from flowers of wild plants and trees, diluted in water. They are similar to homeopathic preparations in that they are energy-based, lacking any molecules of the original material.

Dr Edward Bach, a homeopath working in the 1930s, felt that homeopathy was too preoccupied with the idea of putting things right. In his view illness was a learning process related to a person's greater purpose in life, and true healing came from within. Thus the physical details of an illness were far less important than the false beliefs and negative emotions related to the illness. It is to these factors that the Bach flower remedies are directed. The specific healing properties of each plant were devised intuitively by Dr Bach.

Bach flower remedies are prescribed in much the same way as homeopathic remedies, with a strong emphasis on your psychological and emotional state. The therapist will ask about your illness, especially how you feel about it. This will offer insight into which remedy most resonates with your problem.

The remedies act at the mental body level to free up our access to the causal body. This effect filters down to the emotional, etheric, and finally the physical bodies.

The remedies are useful for all physical conditions and are particularly helpful in conjunction with psychotherapy, as they help to free up changes in consciousness – one of the positive aspects of suffering from any illness. The remedies are good for treating acute illnesses when taken for the few days of the illness. For long-standing illnesses they may need to be continued for months to gain real benefit.

How the remedies are made

The remedies are made from the healthiest flower specimens, picked at their peak. Then they are left outside, steeping in spring water on a sunny day, so the Sun's energy can imprint the water with the flower's energy field. At the end of the day, the water is filtered off and mixed with brandy, which fixes the energy pattern in the water so that it remains stable indefinitely.

ANTHROPOSOPHY

Benefits

Many conditions respond well to the anthroposophical approach, which works well with orthodox medicine. Hayfever, low back pain, and arthritis are very common conditions that are often hard to treat with orthodox methods, but respond well to anthroposophical treatment. General debility, such as with chronic fatigue syndrome, anxiety, and depression, can all benefit from this multi-faceted approach. It also has a respected place in the treatment of cancer.

Anthroposophical medicine is an integrated system of treatments inspired by Rudolf Steiner, who perceived that the human being is made up of physical and subtle energy bodies and that disturbances in any or several of these bodies lead to ill health. He believed that the physical body was enveloped in three layers of subtle bodies, similar to the system described on pages 36–40.

Anthroposophical medicine aims to assess where in the subtle body system an illness originates and which approaches would therefore be best. It includes orthodox diagnoses and treatment and anthroposophical doctors have an initial orthodox medical training. Anthroposophical medicines are prepared similarly to homeopathic remedies, though indications for prescribing may be different from homeopathy. Herbal medicines are often used too, and also physically based treatments, such as hydrotherapy and oil-based massages. Movement therapy, eurythmy (see p. 88), and art therapy are both psychological and spiritual approaches, used along with spiritually based counselling.

You will be asked about your illness, past illness, and treatments, and also about your emotional state and life direction. The examination will focus on what you are like physically (body temperature, build, and posture). X rays or blood tests may be taken if your medical diagnosis is unclear. Then your doctor is likely to prescribe anthroposophical, homeopathic, or herbal preparations to stimulate the etheric body's healing response. Physical treatments, such as massage, may also be prescribed to work at the same level.

Chronic illnesses often need treatment at other levels. Eurythmy, art therapy, and counselling are useful to aid healing and also to provide experiences which may help a person to explore the deeper meaning of their illness and their spiritual nature.

Acute conditions will often only need a single treatment, while chronic illness may benefit from a longer period of treatment.

FENG SHUI

Feng shui is the ancient Chinese study of how to live in accordance with the forces of nature. This study, which is both an art and a science, is over 7000 years old and can be applied to every facet of daily life. In the West, feng shui is gaining popularity as a method of allocating room use, and arranging furniture, plants, and decorations to maximize wellbeing. The Chinese also use it to ensure a harmonious relationship between a building and its environment.

The subtle energies of our environment impinge not only on the physical body but also on the etheric body. Chronic and severe disturbances at a subtle level may ultimately be a cause of illness. Feng shui harnesses these energies for our benefit.

The theories of feng shui enable a practitioner to look at the position of a house, the room use, and the placing of furniture and ornaments in order to ascertain whether the chi flow is healthy or not. He or she looks for places where energy is disrupted or "stuck", or where it may be moving too fast to be of benefit. The consultation involves a survey of the house, sometimes using a feng shui compass to ascertain energies. The flow of chi through the front door and around the rooms, and between the combination of the five elements in decoration and objects is noted. Most attention is paid to the bedrooms, kitchen, and bathroom. As we spend such a proportion of our lives asleep, healthy chi flow in the bedroom is particularly important. The kitchen is where most internal chi is created, as the heat of cooking, while bathrooms are where most chi is lost as waste water draining away.

The consultant will suggest alterations in room use, furniture, and ornament positions, to achieve a balance of chi energy. Sometimes additional objects, such as crystals, wind chimes, or mirrors may be recommended to enhance or neutralize energy patterns. In the following weeks, expect to notice subtle, surprising changes, which may affect how you feel in the house and your health, relationships, and even your "luck", in a positive way.

CLASS 9
Combating negative influences

feng shui
dowsing

Methods that detect, remove, or neutralize damaging energies from our environment. Such environmental energies mainly affect the etheric body. Some can be detected using sensitive scientific instruments, for example, electrical fields. Others, such as underground water, can be detected by dowsing.

The two feng shui schools
The Form school of feng shui bases its understanding of interchange of energies on the principles of the five elements (see p. 45). The Compass school uses the "ba-gua", or feng shui compass, to assess the interchange of energy in any environment, from the layout of a city to the layout of a desk.

DOWSING

Dowsing is a means of detecting and treating geopathic stress, the result of Earth energies that are destructive to health and wellbeing. The Earth has its own aura, or energy fields, and our energy fields have evolved to harmonize with these, helping us to maintain good health. However if the Earth's field becomes distorted, or manmade fields are super-imposed, this harmony can be destroyed, making us feel uncomfortable or even ill.

Many geopathic stresses cannot be detected, but they can be "felt" by sensitives using dowsing methods. In most cases a dowser can detect and treat geopathic stress by inspecting your home and dowsing everywhere, usually using L-shaped rods held in the hands. He or she will look for stresses, taking particular care over beds, favourite chairs, and workplaces. Once detected the stresses can be neutralized or diverted, most commonly by inserting copper rods into the ground, but sometimes by using needles, wooden stakes, crystals, or a small cairn. Normally a single treatment is sufficient.

You may begin to feel the effects of the treatment immediately, although the full benefits will take a few months to manifest. Illnesses triggered by geo-pathic stresses should improve after this time.

Geopathic stress is seen as a contributing factor to many illnesses. Serious illnesses for which no cause is known, such as multiple sclerosis, motor neurone disease, Parkinson's, and Crohn's disease have all been related to it, and cancer seems particularly linked. Chronic fatigue syndrome and multiple allergy and hormonal imbalances, such as PMS, can also be associated with geopathic stress, as can other, less serious, diseases such as minor allergies, recurrent viruses, headaches, migraines, and IBS. Psychological illness and upset such as anxiety, depression, aggression, and hyperactivity are also common reactions. And irritating, non-specific com-plaints such as lethargy, feeling "drained", "on edge", or irritable since moving to a new home can also be caused by geopathic stress.

COLOUR THERAPY

The use of colour for healing is first mentioned in the Vedas (see p. 46), but it is also used in shamanic traditions. Theo Gimbel, inspired by the ideas of Rudolf Steiner, re-established colour as a therapy in the 1950s. Since then colour has gained credibility as a healing tool.

In Gimbel's theory, based on mystical texts, matter is made up of energy and can be considered as "solidified light". Therefore, matter responds to light and in particular responds differently to different wavelengths, or colours, of light.

The colours used in healing are created by shining full-spectrum lighting through high-quality stained glass, producing a rich range in the harmonics of the colour's wavelength. Each individual has a personal wavelength to which he or she responds maximally.

The treatment starts with assessing your spinal column by using a dowsing method on a chart representing the spine. The spine is divided into four sections representing the mental, emotional, metabolic, and physical bodies. Within each section are eight vertebrae, each with the energies of one colour from the therapy spectrum. The spectrum is based on four pairs of complementary colours. The therapist dowses to find which colour energies are active in your spine, colouring in the spine chart with the appropriate colours.

Each coloured vertebra is then paired with its complementary elsewhere on the chart. The unpaired colour is the one that is out of balance in your body and is the one used in your therapy. Wearing white clothes, you are bathed in this colour, and then with its complementary. The colours are shone though shapes associated with them, which also complement each other.

Treatments take time for the body to assimilate and the usual interval between sessions is three to four weeks. Three treatments are usually sufficient. Between times you may be advised to wear "your" colour and occasionally its complementary. You may also be asked to use these colours in a visualization.

CLASS 10
Enhancing positive energies

colour therapy
sound therapy

These are methods of physically shaping our environment, which affects us through our senses. The senses have a strong effect on the emotional body.

Colour healing

Colours can be used more informally in healing, by changing the colours you wear, your work or home colour schemes, or using visualizations or movements to enhance your experience of a colour that benefits you.

SOUND THERAPY

Sound as a healing tool dates from the earliest days of healing practices – the shamanic traditions. These use single notes from bells, cymbals, bowls, and didgeridoos and also repetitive chants and rhythms from drums and rattles, which are all seen to have spiritual as well as healing purposes.

Benefits

Psychological conditions, such as depression and anxiety, respond well to sound therapy and it can help relieve the stress of chronic illness. It has a particular function as a health maintenance tool that combines creativity, fun, and sharing with the subtle effects that sound has on the physical and energy bodies.

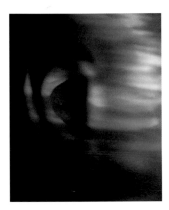

The present revival in sound therapy probably began with Rudolf Steiner, who combined it with movement in eurythmy (see p. 88). Its popularity grew further in the 1960s and 1970s, with the increased interest in shamanism and energy healing.

Sound is not just related to hearing; the vibrations that create it are also picked up by the rest of the body. Indeed we can feel some low-frequency sounds in our bodies although we cannot hear them. In energy healing this vibration is considered to affect the various subtle bodies, especially the emotions. The chakras (see pp. 46–9) are very sensitive to the effects of sound, as are the meridians in Traditional Chinese Medicine (see p. 44).

Some sound therapists work with individual patients to treat specific problems with sound. Others concentrate on group work, which has less specific goals but allows everyone to participate in mutual healing.

Sound therapies use sound in a number of ways, often in combination. Musical techniques include chanting (singing repetitive songs) or toning (playing or singing single, often prolonged, notes). Participants may also listen to rhythms, or create their own. Sometimes more complex music is played or listened to. In addition, sound therapy can also include the making of "natural" sounds such as laughter or sighing.

Sound therapy, whether practised alone or in a group, is both energizing and relaxing. It also helps us get in touch with and express our emotions, making it a very good technique for stress management. Making sounds or music together rapidly brings cohesiveness to a group and this helps us to feel connected to others.

JUNGIAN PSYCHOANALYSIS

Psychoanalysis was originally developed by Sigmund Freud in the 1890s and Carl Jung (1865–1961) is probably the most well known of his followers.

Jung was aware of the subtle bodies and this technique seems to work primarily on the mental body, through which it accesses the emotional and etheric bodies. It also contacts the causal body.

The first two sessions are likely to be devoted to finding out what has brought you to analysis and assessing your expectations, goals, and needs. You will agree a verbal contract, setting out for how long and how often you will attend. This is usually a minimum of two years of two to four sessions a week. Obviously this is a huge commitment, so it is important to be sure that you recognize that your original problem or illness is a way to start exploring your unconscious – a journey into the unknown.

Analysis is not simply a method of getting rid of your problem or illness. You will find yourself initiating the talking and you will do most of it. You are free to talk about whatever you like, and your analyst will not interfere with your progression of thought. By this means the unconscious is slowly opened up and explored. The therapist may encourage a deepening of your experience by asking you to expand on certain points. He or she may offer an interpretation of what you talk about. During the process "transference" to the therapist usually occurs; identifying him or her with an important person, such as your father, mother, or ideal lover. Unresolved feelings can thus be worked through as the process unfolds.

Jungian analysis can point the way to a greater understanding of yourself. It is not simply about problem-solving, but a spiritual quest for a meaning to life. However, psychosomatically and psychologically based illnesses are often relieved during the analysis. Major psychological illnesses, such as schizophrenia or bipolar affective disorder (BAD), can be helped by this approach, but should not be treated without medical supervision.

CLASS 11
Psychology

Jungian psychoanalysis
hypnotherapy
neurolinguistic
    programming
autogenic training
re-evaluation counselling
shamanic healing

These methods use the mind. Different techniques have effects on different energy bodies. For example, relaxation techniques primarily affect the etheric body.

Theory

Analysis primarily allows us to delve deep into our own sense of being, giving insight into how we respond to others and how we function as well as connecting us more closely with the Self.

According to the Jungian approach, our normal waking state is called our consciousness and the part of our mind, or psyche, of which we are not normally aware, our unconsciousness. The unconscious part is what gives us difficulties, such as illnesses or relationship problems, and is always at work.

HYPNOTHERAPY

Benefits

Hypnotherapy can help a wide number of conditions and medication will not impede its effectiveness. Psychological problems and psychosomatic illness are especially responsive, but other physical illnesses, such as chronic illness and cancer, may respond well. It is an excellent way of dealing with the stress that can cause, and is produced by, any illness. Hypnosis is also used very successfully in the treatment of addictions and for pain control.

This form of psychotherapy uses hypnosis to access the subconscious by inducing deep relaxation. It uses the mental body to access the emotional body, which can help to change belief patterns that may underlie psychological illness. Changes in the emotional body can also filter down to the etheric and physical bodies and lead to an improved sense of wellbeing.

Sessions are usually weekly and last about one hour. The first concentrates on problems, physical and psychological, and lifestyle information.

There are many ways in which hypnosis can be "induced", but for all of them it is important that you trust the therapist and are willing to suspend disbelief. A common method is to ask you to focus on a point above your natural sight line and breathe slowly. As you relax you watch as the therapist draws his or her thumb from the bridge of your nose up to the middle of your forehead, while you roll your eyes upward and imagine a peaceful scene. The therapist then counts from ten to one, asking you to relax deeper on each count. On "one" you are asked to let go of all tension. By this stage the access to the subconscious mind is made, although your consciousness can override unacceptable suggestions and you are always in control.

The therapist will make suggestions to your subconscious to boost confidence, self-worth, and wellbeing. The next stage is to use this access to your subconscious to change old beliefs and patterns, by allowing you to re-examine what triggered them and to replace them with more appropriate beliefs about yourself.

Closing the session will include suggestions to your subconscious that you will feel better in yourself, more confident, and that the process started in the subconscious will continue as you move back to normality. He or she will then bring you out of hypnosis by asking you to visualize a pleasant image and then, after a count of seven, to return to waking consciousness, feeling alert, relaxed, and hopeful.

WARNING

Serious psychological illness such as depression, schizophrenia, and bipolar affective disorder (BAD) need particular expertise and should not be treated without full medical supervision.

NEUROLINGUISTIC PROGRAMMING

This psychotherapeutic technique (NLP for short) is designed to help you understand how you think and feel, thus enabling you to make new choices about how you respond to your circumstances. NLP considers that we all have the answer to any of life's problems. Our difficulty is in accessing this and NLP offers a way.

The first step is to discover whether you think in a visual, auditory, or kinesthetic manner. The next is to reorientate your own perception of your problem. This is done by carrying out mental exercises to reveal your thought processes and then to offer you alternative ways of thinking.

A number of techniques can be used. You may be encouraged to trace your ideas about the problem to a behaviour pattern that may no longer be appropriate. For example, you may have coped with authority as a child by avoiding it, and this has become a pattern. The process of "reframing" allows you to change the way you feel about the problem and often leads to the solution. This is greatly empowering – in itself healing.

The techniques can be applied not only to health problems but also to work, relationships, and the "inner struggle", which is often tied to physical illness. NLP works primarily on the belief system and therefore on the mental body. Changing beliefs also tends to connect us more directly to the causal body. These changes filter down to influence our emotional, etheric, and physical bodies.

An NLP practitioner may ask about your basic problem. As you talk he or she will watch your body language, including the way you speak and use words, breathing patterns, and eye movements. This gives insight into your personal way of processing thought and emotion.

Ideally an NLP session is open-ended, going on to a point of resolution, but even if the problem is not solved, it may be "reframed" better. After the session your mind will continue working with the new approach and further changes may happen.

Origins

NLP was developed in the 1970s by Americans Richard Bandler and John Grinder, who studied how a group of successful therapists worked. They discovered that the way these approached the processing of thought and emotion was their key to success. Bandler and Grinder analyzed this processing into its components and translated it into the NLP technique.

Benefits

NLP is designed to move problems on quickly, so effects should be experienced after a few sessions. This is especially true for the treatment of specific conditions such as phobias, for which it is very effective. It is also good for breaking mental habits, such as smoking, and for enabling us to make better life choices, such as how we are in our relationships.

AUTOGENIC TRAINING

Benefits

AT is of great help in chronic conditions, psychosomatic elements of illness, and psychological upset. Headaches and migraines are responsive and asthma is particularly so – the technique can help prevent or limit acute attacks. High blood pressure, irritable bowel syndrome, insomnia, bladder disorders, arthritis, and even diabetes and AIDS are all conditions that have been helped by AT.

Regular practitioners suffer fewer acute illnesses, such as viruses, which is some evidence that AT boosts the functioning of the immune system. It is also good for psychological states such as phobias, panic attacks, irritability, and anxiety.

Autogenic training (AT) is a psychotherapeutically based self-help tool, combining some elements of meditation with relaxation and affirmation.

AT is thought to work by balancing the activities of the left (dominant) and right (passive) sides of the brain. This helps to restore emotional balance and has beneficial effects on the autonomic, or unconscious, aspect of the nervous system, which plays a part in many physical illnesses.

AT theory does not relate to the theories of subtle bodies, but the technique appears to have powerful effects on the emotional and mental bodies. This filters down to the etheric and physical bodies, alleviating symptoms. It also acts in the same way as meditation to improve the connection to the causal body. This relieves stress, as it allows us to connect more closely to the part of ourselves that exists beyond the stresses of everyday life.

AT is taught mainly by doctors, nurses, or other healthcare professionals, who have learned it in addition to their original training. It is usually taught in groups of six to eight people, although sometimes individual lessons are more appropriate.

Before you start group sessions you will have an assessment. There are some conditions, such as schizophrenia and severe mental illness, in which AT is not appropriate, and other conditions, such as heart disease, where the methods may need to be modified. The sessions themselves are one and a half hours long and take place over eight to ten weeks. In them you learn the six standard exercises: heaviness of the limbs; warmth in the limbs; focusing on the heartbeat; breathing; warmth in the abdomen, and coolness in the forehead. You will be expected to keep a diary of your sessions and to practise for up to ten minutes three times a day. Other techniques, such as personal and motivational formulae (positive affirmations) and intentional exercises may be introduced. All the exercises need to be undertaken with a passive concentration, without trying or expecting results, but noting what is happening.

RE-EVALUATION COUNSELLING

Re-evaluation counselling (RC) is a psychological tool in which there is no hierarchy between therapist and client. In an RC course you learn to be both, and have sessions with a partner from the course where you can divide the time in each role equally between you.

The RC technique was developed in the 1950s in America by Harvey Jackins, whose theory of human behaviour proposed that difficulties we have in coping stem from irrational behaviour patterns, triggered by an inappropriate emotional response to a situation. For example, suppose that as a child you are confronted with a problem and become upset. If instead of being able to enter fully into the experience you are told to be quiet or are placated, this stops the complete "discharge" of the emotion. Then, whenever a similar situation occurs, your normal spontaneous problem-solving mechanism is over-ridden by re-stimulation of the old distress. As you are now programmed that it is unacceptable to enter into distress and so "discharge" it, you repress its expression yet again, and so the cycle is primed to continue.

Some of these distresses are so often activated that they become permanently stimulated. This leads to what seem to be difficult personality traits, while they are really chronic irrational responses that could be cleared. The primary purpose of RC is to recover your capacity to think and to react more rationally, rather than as a response to old distresses.

RC works at the level of the emotional and mental bodies to clear distress patterns held in the emotional body that influence the mental body. The effects of this distress can filter down to the physical level and appear as psychosomatic illness.

RC is essentially a training. A basic course usually consists of weekly and weekend sessions and between sessions you practise with a partner from the course. Afterward you are eligible to exchange counselling sessions with others trained in RC, also known as "co-counselling".

Benefits
RC is particularly good for psychological problems and may also help reduce the psychosomatic component of an illness. It is also a good means of support in chronic or terminal illness in that it helps to process associated feelings.

The discharge process
Discharge is the spontaneous release of an emotion such as laughter or tears or the release at a physical level such as shuddering or yawning. Once the discharge begins it is important that it is allowed to continue until it finds its natural resolution. This starts the process of releasing the client from the stuck, irrational responses that they formerly held.

SHAMANIC HEALING

Benefits

Shamanic healing is used particularly to help psychological problems, which may also be tied in with a physical ailment.

It is also notably helpful for hormonal problems, especially thyroid, and female hormone upsets, such as heavy menstruation, and the menopause and its symptoms. Shamanic healing complements other methods of healing, especially orthodox treatments.

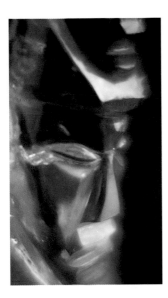

Shamanism is by far the most ancient healing tradition, at least 50,000 years old. The shamanic view of the cosmos is animistic: everything in the Universe is alive and therefore has a spirit, which in some cases can detach from its physical form. It is this "free spirit" form that is used in shamanic trance states, or "journeying".

Even thoughts and emotions are considered to have a spirit component. One of the causes of illness is the "spirit" of the illness coming into our "spirit" body and affecting the physical body.

Modern shamanic healing is an adaptation of ancient traditional forms of healing, the work of shamans and medicine men and women. Intrinsic to this form of healing is the use of ritual and altered states of awareness. In so-called primitive cultures shamanism is generally respected more than orthodox Western medicine.

Traditional shamanic healing uses herbal preparations in two ways: to treat the patient and to induce altered states of consciousness in the shaman. This latter use is discouraged in present-day Westernized shamanism.

According to shamanism, illness can happen in a number of ways; one of the most common is as a result of "soul loss". This occurs because of trauma, which may be physical or emotional and may precede the illness by years. The shock of the trauma causes part of our spirit body to leave and the "hole" becomes filled by the spirit of an illness. In a shamanic healing the shaman uses his free spirit form as well as enlisting the help of a spirit guide, "power animals", or "spirit helper". Together they persuade the spirit of the illness to leave.

For the treatment the shaman is in a trance, which enables him or her to enter the spirit world. Western civilization today would see this as a type of creative visualization, but the world of the shaman is said to be more "real" than simple imagination. The treatment may help at the physical and emotional levels or in the other subtle bodies.

PRAYER

Prayer is normally considered in a religious context, which is where it originated. It is an ancient way of expressing thankfulness or asking for help from that which is beyond everyday life. It has much in common with affirmation (see p. 40), although its potential for results is higher, since intent is directed to the most subtle of our connections to universal consciousness, often referred to as "God". This aligns the emotional and mental bodies to the causal body, and the effect can filter down through the etheric to the physical bodies, sometimes creating miraculous changes, including healing.

Words used in prayer are important. In ancient religious traditions, such as Hebrew and Sanskrit, not only the words themselves but also their sound and the way they are written are important for their power. Words and sounds are considered to come from a divine source. The Bible refers to this ancient power of the word, which has become diminished since humans have taken words for their own use. Most of our languages come from an Indo-European source, of which Hebrew and Sanskrit are the most ancient examples, so our present-day languages do still carry divine sounds.

The wording of a prayer may follow tradition. For example the Christian Lord's Prayer is well known and oft-repeated. This repetition, through populations and generations, increases its subtle energies. However, without understanding and feeling much of the potency of the prayer is lost.

Prayers can also be used for protection. Religious people often repeat prayers of invocation during ordeals. Sacred texts or symbols are also used in this way to protect houses – Orthodox Jews fix scrolls of text to their doorposts. A short prayer repeated continuously can also be used for meditation; in Sanskrit this is known as a "mantra". The use of rosaries in Catholicism and prayer wheels in Buddhism are other examples of this use of prayer. For effectiveness these need to be used with focus and intent and not as absent-minded repetition.

CLASS 12
Meditation

prayer
meditation

These are mental techniques that you have to practise and whose effects are cumulative. Physically you need to maintain a wakeful position and consciousness of breathing. Meditation methods have the potential to affect all the energy bodies and ultimately establish a connection between the causal body and "divine" states beyond.

Types of prayer

Invocation is an earnest request, for example, for a return to health. It is made to whatever energy beyond the Self the person believes in and is a connection with the causal body and beyond.

A prayer of thankfulness aligns the emotional, mental, and causal bodies. It is a kind of surrender and can open up the subtle bodies to healing energies beyond the Self.

MEDITATION

Benefits

Meditation helps people cope with stress and so is good for anxiety and psychosomatic illnesses. It is also good in recovery from addictions and has been found useful in convalescence from heart disease and as an aid to insomnia. Sufferers of terminal or chronic disease can also benefit.

Meditation should be avoided by sufferers of depression, schizophrenia, or bipolar affective disorder (BAD), unless the symptoms are under control, and a supportive teacher is available, in which case it can be of great benefit.

Meditation positions

Traditional schools, such as yoga and Buddhism, consider that the pose itself influences meditation. For example, in hatha yoga the full lotus is believed to benefit meditation. But some Western schools consider that contact with the Earth through the feet, while sitting in an upright chair, maximizes meditation effects. Most schools consider that lying down is not good. There are also walking meditations, where slow walking is used as the seed or focus.

There are also different ways of using the eyes: closed, semi-closed, or open with soft focus. Different hand positions may also be recommended. In hatha yoga these "mudras" are used specifically to affect states of consciousness.

Meditation is a discipline, not a therapy, with the potential to heal at all levels. It is a way of using thought to relax body and mind and can open up awareness of different states of consciousness. Practised for over 4000 years, it is mentioned in the Vedas and is an integral part of yoga. It is also important in religions, particularly Buddhism.

Meditation is a way of controlling thought processes and body function, allowing a new way of perceiving consciousness. The process is designed to move consciousness beyond the ego. Meditation can take us beyond bodily discomforts, stopping the "busy-ness" of our minds, beyond our sense of ourselves to one where we feel bliss, one-ness with the "divine", joy, peace, and a rightness about life. The underlying theory is that beyond our everyday mind there is a richer realm, where our ordinary sense of who we are and our purpose in life becomes eclipsed by a greater sense of reality. Meditation is a way of opening to our causal body, and also to that which lies beyond. In order to experience this our other subtle bodies and our physical body have to come into closer alignment.

There are two main styles of meditation: "no-mind" and "seed". In "no-mind", thoughts, images, or emotions pass without reaction from the ego. Eventually these distractions stop arising and a state of emptiness is experienced. This can be filled with a profound joy, love, or bliss – a feeling of being connected to everything – the state of "samadi", or enlightenment. In "seed" meditation there is focus for the ego, such as the breath, a candle, a word, an image, or a phrase, usually sacred, such as a mantra. Thoughts and feelings that arise are not given attention – but the attention to the focus is increased. Seed is considered by some to be more effective as the ego mind is designed to focus on something and asking it not to is artificial. Once the ego mind has a focus the inner mind is free to expand to fill our sense of awareness. Both forms of meditation can produce the experience of enlightenment.

When you begin meditating, start with ten minutes, at regular times (for example, morning and evening), in a special place. Gradually build up the time to around thirty minutes.

Meditation has both immediate and long-term benefits. Immediate benefits include relaxation, serenity, peace, joy, and love, together with a sense of energy flowing though your body, connectedness to everything, and a sense of being in touch with the "divine". Longer-term benefits include wellbeing, emotional equilibrium, and transformation of negative emotions into love, awareness, greater compassion, a deeper sense of purpose or direction, and a sense of the bigger picture.

A common disturbance is the mind racing. This can be counteracted by focusing more attentively on the seed or just letting the process run on for a few minutes. Try not to force thoughts or emotions to stop – just gently let them go. Another problem is physical discomfort. If you have chosen the wrong position, change it. Try focusing with more concentration on your seed, or else focus briefly on the pain – it will usually transform into a relaxed state.

Occasionally you may feel disturbed. This is probably because you are opening up your subtle bodies, so that you are either experiencing previously suppressed emotions or sensations, or else your openness is exposing you to thoughts or emotions belonging to all humanity. If you stay focused on your seed this helps release the disturbance, and you should move beyond it. If not, come out of the meditation, eat or drink something, and do something active. If this is a recurrent problem, only continue meditating with a group or teacher to support you until you pass through this stage.

All meditators go through periods of loss of interest, lack of progress, or even regression. This is temporary and you should attempt to continue your routine. Some people use meditation to escape from life's reality and spend too long in it. This is a serious trap: if it happens, stop meditating and consult your teacher, doctor, or psychotherapist.

Meditation on the breath
This is a widely practised form of seed meditation.
• Find a comfortable position, focus your attention within, on your breath. Watch and feel it coming in and out of your lungs. Do not force your breath in or out, and don't interfere with the rests between inspiration and expiration.

• Concentrate on your breathing and let thoughts pass without becoming distracted. After a while you may find that you are not breathing but being "breathed". This indicates a different state of consciousness.

Images in meditation
Physical images can be used as a focus or seed. The most well-known is the "yantra" – a mandala designed to encourage a specific state of consciousness, for example opening the heart chakra. Tibetan Buddhism uses sacred images of gods and goddesses, each of which elicits different states of consciousness. The use of icons in Christianity has a similar function. In secular forms of meditation, beautiful images or objects, especially those from nature, may be used.

CLASS 13

Power objects

talismans
crystal healing

Talismans and crystals have a similar effect to meditation. They are often used to enhance healing methods as they seem to boost both the therapist's and the client's capacity to make effective changes in the energy bodies.

Children's special objects

Children naturally give certain objects special significance, for example their favourite soft toy or blanket. This is an example of our innate tendency to imbue objects with power.

TALISMANS

A talisman is an object that confers protection from negative energies; it is a "lucky charm". It can also act as a focus of intent to intensify meditation, prayer, or healing. Religious icons and holy objects have similar functions, and so can objects from nature such as crystals, rocks, shells, or pieces of wood. Objects worn at a time of good fortune or received from a highly respected person can also be imbued with protective or supportive qualities.

The energy field of a talisman comes from its source. Power objects from nature carry the innate healing, grounding energy of nature, which the user can tap into when their own energy fields are disturbed. Talismans from a religious source should be made by devotees of the religion or blessed by a priest or equivalent. This aligns the talisman and its energy field to the "divine" or universal consciousness. In addition, using a talisman for meditation or prayer intensifies its energy field. Tapping into this field by holding or focusing on the object further aids the ability to meditate or pray. The use of the Jewish tallis prayer shawl and the Islamic prayer mat exploits this property.

A talisman has a psychological effect and in this way can influence the emotional and mental bodies, but it seems to affect connection to the causal body and to universal consciousness or the "divine". A person may outgrow the need for a talisman. This happens when the person's consciousness and their connection to their subtle bodies has shifted, so that there is no longer a need for an external focus.

Any object that is to be used as a talisman needs to come from a reliable source that has imbued it with only the most subtle energies. If you are not sure of the source, cleanse it as you would a crystal (see p. 112). You should not use a talisman for a variety of purposes as this will dissipate energy. A talisman belonging to another, or from childhood, does not carry such fine energies and its effect is psychological. However, as long as its use is not obsessive it can be of value.

CRYSTAL HEALING

Crystals have been used as healing tools for thousands of years, especially in shamanic healing – one of the oldest healing traditions. Since the 1960s, crystals have experienced an upsurge in popularity as healing tools, in meditation, and in rituals.

The simple, but exact, internal order of crystals seems to be important to healing function, making them into a kind of natural hologram. They also contain energy, though in stable form. These crystal properties are used in technology, for example in quartz clocks, where exact time-keeping is the result of energy being released when the crystal is stressed.

A belief shared by many healers is that the crystal acts as a natural "tuning fork", to which the human energy field resonates. If our energy bodies are "out of tune" because of disease the crystal helps restore harmony by bringing them into line with the crystal's vibration.

The clear focus of energy that crystals provide enhances our ability to work with the subtle energies. Crystals seem to have a particularly potent effect on the emotional body, from which they can affect the etheric and physical body and release the mental body to align with the causal body.

A crystal healer will ask about medical problems, your emotional state and life stresses, and what you hope to receive. Finally, you may be asked to choose a crystal to which you are intuitively drawn. We are naturally attracted to those crystals whose energy pattern we can most benefit from.

The session starts with an exercise to help you relax. Next you may be asked to hold the crystals and have them placed on your body, most likely over the chakras. Others may be placed around your body. The therapist may then move a crystal around your body, but not touching, to direct healing to your subtle bodies. You may feel tingling, warmth, coolness, expansion, or pressure and you may also experience emotional reactions. Overall, the session is relaxing, and you may fall into a dreamlike state, or sleep.

Cleansing crystals
To rid crystals of negative emotional energies cleanse them regularly, especially if they are used for healing or exposed to strong emotions. Whatever method you use, carry out the ritual with love and the intent to cleanse all that is extraneous to the crystal's natural vibration.

• Wash them in flowing water and leave them to air-dry.

• Leave them outside on the earth for 24 hours.

• Use mental cleansing methods such as visualization or prayer.

Benefits
Crystal healing is excellent for stress relief and emotional problems. It is therefore very helpful for illnesses with a psychosomatic component such as headaches, migraines, IBS, indigestion, and asthma. The healing can be applied not only to the human body but also to our environment – at home or in the workplace. Crystal healing techniques are used in feng shui (see p. 98) and in the reduction of geopathic stress (see p. 99).

Methods that are apparently physical, whose underlying philosophies are based on concepts of body energy systems. Their treatments have both a physical and an energetic component.

The five elements and their qualities

ETHER = *minuteness*

AIR = *lightness, mobility, and roughness*

FIRE = *hotness, lightness, and sharpness*

WATER = *coolness, liquidity, softness, smoothness*

EARTH = *heaviness, solidity, stability*

Benefits

Ayurvedic medicine can be used to treat any illness, but it is particularly good for chronic and psychosomatic illnesses. It is especially helpful in illnesses that cannot be treated successfully by orthodox medicine, for example irritable bowel syndrome, chronic fatigue syndrome, and pre-menstrual tension.

AYURVEDIC MEDICINE

Ayurvedic medicine, developed in India 5000 years ago, is a complete system of healing, drawing together all aspects of life and relating them to health and wellbeing. Based on ancient tradition, it considers everything in the Universe to be made of varying combinations of five "elements" (see below left). From observation of the world it is possible to detect the balance of the five elements present.

In ayurvedic medicine, illness is seen as an upset in the balance of energies within the body. The mind, emotions, and physical levels of being are considered to be inextricably linked and are influenced by the activities of three life-giving energies known as "doshas" – Vatta (V), Kapha (K), and Pitta (P) (see p. 114). Each dosha is made up of two of the five elements. The words used to describe the concepts of elements and doshas are attempts to describe the feeling that the definitions convey. To understand them you need to explore how you experience them and how each feels relative to another in your body and mind.

Each person is born with an inherited physical constitution. Most people have one dominant or, less commonly, a mixture of two, equally dominant, doshas. Your dominant dosha determines the features that make you unique, such as your hair colour, body shape, and the kinds of foods you tend to crave, and also they signify the type of illness from which you are most likely to suffer. The balance between the doshas, according to your constitutional mix, is most important for the maintenance of health. Throughout a life-time this mixture varies a little, even in health. For example, childhood is more K, adulthood is more P, and old age is more V.

Our environment also influences the proportions of the doshas. The climate, season, and colours of clothes or in the home are just some factors that can all have an effect. In health we can adjust to these constantly varying influences, but in illness our own proportions are out of balance and these environmental influences can worsen the situation.

Our dominant dosha type tends to draw us to experiences in the environment that stimulate this dosha ("like attracting like"). Thus we can find ourselves in a lifestyle that overstimulates our predominant dosha, leading to ill health. To correct this we need to make lifestyle changes to pacify the overactive dosha and incorporate more of the doshas we lack. This restores constitutional balance and health by changing the environmental influences to aid our internal balance.

Ayurveda particularly concentrates on diet, considering that food, cooking methods, food combinations, and timing of meals all affect the balance of doshas. Every foodstuff inherently has either a stimulating or pacifying effect on each dosha, and we tend to be attracted to foods that stimulate our dominant dosha. A major part of an ayurvedic treatment is assessing what foods are appropriate to pacify the dosha whose excess has led to ill health.

An ayurvedic doctor also uses herbs medicinally to increase the pacification of the dosha when dietary changes are insufficient. Since ayurveda recognizes the importance of the emotional state and also our deep beliefs and spiritual attitudes, meditation may also be recommended to balance the doshas at these levels.

A consultation consists of an interview, where the practitioner assesses how your illness affects each level of your subtle bodies. Your original constitutional dosha will be considered, plus your daily routine, work, leisure, digestion, sleep, and, most importantly, diet. There will also be a physical examination. Next the therapist will draw up a programme of dietary modification and lifestyle changes, such as changes in routines, minimizing the dosha-enhancing effects of your work, leisure pursuits, room and clothing colours. These changes should be incorporated in stages, to work gradually toward restoring the constitutional balance of the doshas. In addition, your practitioner may recommend oiling and massage, and give advice on meditation and ways of releasing old emotions.

Examples of dosha characteristics

VATTA

- *Physically thin, overactive, exhausts easily, chilly, rarely sweats.*

- *Emotionally changeable, tends to fears, anxiety, insecurity.*

- *Full of ideas, creative but not proactive.*

- *Has superficial and changeable spiritual beliefs. "Airy" at every level of being.*

PITTA

- *Medium build, manages energy levels well, warm, sweats easily.*

- *Steady moods, but prone to anger, tendency to be judgmental.*

- *Mentally ambitious, competitive, intellectual, good at carrying things through.*

- *Deep spiritual beliefs. "Fiery" at every level of being.*

KAPHA

- *Fat or of heavy build, lazy but has good stamina, cold, tends to sweat.*

- *Emotionally tends to be greedy and possessive, but calm and caring.*

- *A slow thinker but can organize well.*

- *Spiritually holds deep and unchangeable beliefs. "Watery" at every level of being.*

NATUROPATHY

Details of treatments

• DIET – *individually tailored, based on organic, raw wholefoods, with limited animal proteins. Foods are eaten in combinations, allowing maximum absorption of nutrients.*

• SUPPLEMENTS – *vitamin and mineral supplements, herbs, and tissue salts.*

• EXERCISES – *including regular walking or swimming to increase stamina, and stretches to increase flexibility.*

• STRESS MANAGEMENT – *including relaxation exercises, visualizations, and affirmations and ways to approach life in a less stressful way.*

• MANIPULATION – *may be done if the spine is out of alignment.*

• HYDROTHERAPY – *includes sitz baths, cold and warm compresses, wrapping the body in damp sheets, and high-pressure showers.*

Naturopathy incorporates a number of different healing methods that aim to restore our natural state of good health and sense of wellbeing. All are designed to maximize available life force and to teach us how to take control of our health by increasing our understanding of the body and how we can work constructively with it. Naturopathy is strongly based on the idea of wholeness and does not focus on the disease.

Naturopathy was developed in its present form from the work done in the 1890s by the American Dr Lindlahr, and by Dr Bircher-Benner in Europe. However it is rooted in Ancient Greece, with Hippocrates' ideas of health and wellbeing.

Naturopaths believe that disease is an expression of abnormality in the body and that all abnormalities are created by an interference with the body's natural function. Such abnormalities obstruct the flow of the life force, reducing the amount of energy left for living. The obstruction can be at any, or several, levels of our physical and subtle bodies and different naturopathic treatments deal with problems or obstructions at different levels.

In a detailed consultation, your practitioner will ask about your health, medication, diet, and lifestyle. There is also a physical examination. In the second part of the consultation treatments are prescribed. The main focus of treatment is diet, supplements, or remedies, and a psycho-spiritual approach including relaxation and attitudinal changes. Most naturopaths are also osteopaths, and so posture adjustment and advice is also given. Hydrotherapy techniques, such as sitz baths, are also often used.

Naturopathy is useful for conditions where the immune system seems to be malfunctioning, such as allergies, chronic fatigue syndrome, and rheumatoid arthritis. It can also be useful in conjunction with orthodox treatments in the treatment of cancer, as it helps both the patient as a whole, and with the side effects of radiation and chemotherapy.

HERBALISM

This system of healing based on the use of herbs is an ancient healing method. Herbal treatments mainly affect the physical body, and by that route have effects on the other bodies, especially the emotional. These effects at subtle levels appear to be slowly accumulative. All traditional shamanic cultures have used herbalism for healing, and for accessing psychic powers and spiritual experiences.

There is no doubt that herbs have a physiological balancing effect on the metabolism. Orthodox medicine, originally developed from herbalism, has stimulating or suppressing effects.

In a consultation, a herbalist will try to develop a rapport between you in order to build up knowledge about you, your illness, past health problems, and your lifestyle, including your response to stress and diet. There may also be a physical examination. Medical herbalists are sufficiently trained to assess whether you need to see an orthodox doctor first.

You will then be prescribed a course of treatment, which will include dietary advice. There is an over-lap between food and herbs in that all foods affect metabolism and therefore can physically influence an illness. The herbs may be given as tinctures, liquid extracts, or as dried herbs which can be made up into infusions or teas. A prescription usually contains between three and six herbs and is taken three times a day for some weeks. Supplements, such as special foods, for example wheatgerm, and vitamins and minerals, may also be prescribed.

The initial consultation is about an hour long; follow-up sessions, two or three weeks later, usually last half an hour. With time, follow-up sessions become further apart.

Herbalism is suitable for a range of conditions. It can be very effective in acute conditions such as injuries or infections, but it is also very useful for chronic conditions, where its benefits accumulate slowly. Menopausal disorders, stress-related conditions, and digestive problems are especially amenable to herbal treatment.

Animals and herbs
Herbalism probably predates humankind as there are animals, such as the snake, the wolf, and the chimpanzee, who eat herbs when they are ill. This suggests that the choosing of plants for their healing capacity is innate in animals.

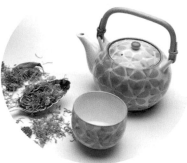

Differing theories
Herbalists differ in their approach. Some take a materialistic, scientific approach, which sees the effects of herbs as entirely biological. Some see the physical effects as being a stimulus to changes at other levels. Others see herbs as having a subtle energy field of their own which interacts with the body's subtle fields. Traditional views of herbalism, which link herbs to astrology and alchemy, certainly considered the herbs to have effects beyond the physical.

CHINESE HERBALISM

Chinese herbalism is one of the key aspects of Traditional Chinese Medicine (see pp. 42–6).

In Traditional Chinese Medicine theory, illness is a disturbance to the flow of life energy, chi, through the body. Although herbs have a physical effect on the body, just as orthodox drugs do, Chinese herbalism has a different concept of these. Their primary effect is seen as modifying and bringing back into balance the flow of chi. Therefore they are seen as therapeutic tools used to restore a healthy balance of energy.

At a consultation you will be questioned about your health problems and lifestyle, especially diet. You may be asked how you are affected by weather or the time of year. Your practitioner will examine you, taking note of your tongue and pulse. From this information a diagnosis can be made. You will probably be given some dietary guidelines to follow, since diet, in conjunction with the herbs, helps to maximize their effectiveness.

Chinese herbal treatments consist of well-tried mixtures of herbs. These may be given in the traditional way, as loose herbs, which you make into a tea, although some practitioners use capsules. The medicines are usually taken several times a day for several weeks, after which the treatment is reviewed. The length of treatment needed varies considerably. Generally, long-standing conditions take longer to respond.

In China and the West there is particular interest in studying the physical or biochemical effects of the preparations as well as their energy effects. Increasingly, evidence suggests that the preparations are useful in the treatment of many ailments. Chinese herbalism can be used to treat a wide range of disorders, but it seems particularly effective for psoriasis, eczema, asthma, digestive problems, and menstrual problems. It has also been found to be useful in the amelioration of the side effects of cancer chemotherapy – an excellent example of complementary medicine in action.

Systems of diagnosis

A TCM diagnosis is different from a Western medical diagnosis, because the two specialities look at the cause of illness very differently. For example, Western medicine sees psoriasis as a single illness to be treated with the same range of drugs. In Chinese medicine psoriasis is differentiated into individualized types with differing causes responding to different herbs. Also Western medicine labels illnesses according to their symptoms, while Chinese medicine names them according to their causes. For example, a Western doctor might see asthma and psoriasis as different diseases needing different treatments, while in Chinese medicine certain cases of asthma and psoriasis have the same cause and therefore need the same treatment.

Part 3

Flow charts for common ailments

The charts in Part Three are designed to enable you to gain deeper insight into your illness and to lead you to classes of therapies (found in Part Two) which are most appropriate to your own healing process. The charts also give information about standard orthodox treatments that are routinely used. By combining the information from this section with information from Part Two, you can draw up a personal plan for healing based on all the available information.

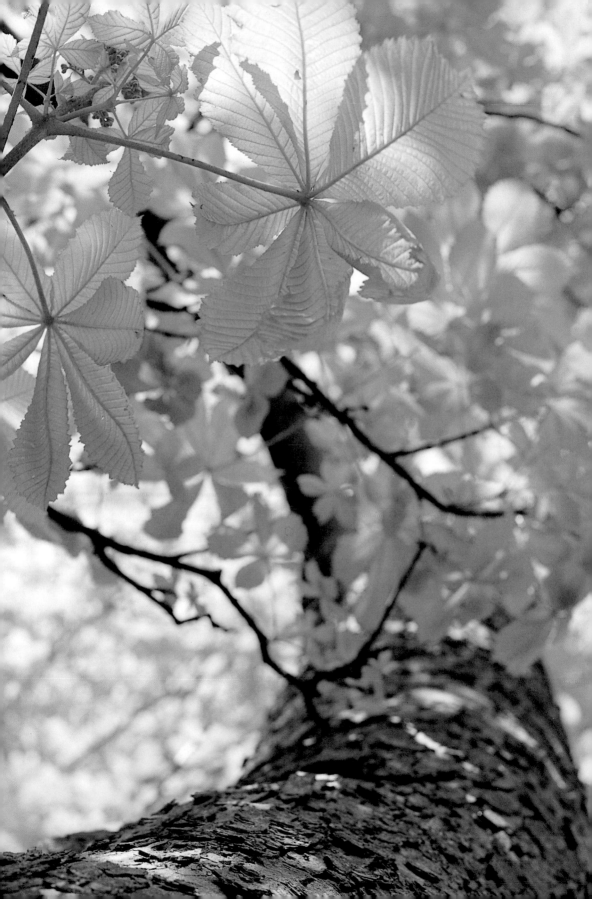

ASTHMA

①

Is your asthma triggered by colds, dust, pollens, animal hair, or feathers?

▶ NO ▶

②

Is your asthma worsened by stress?

▶ NO ▶

③

Did your asthma start early in life (aged 2–5)?

▶ NO ▶ ▶ ▶

▼
YES
▼

There is a fault in the working of your immune system, the most physical part of the innate self-healing mechanism. To correct its malfunction all the energy bodies may need assistance.
Consult a therapist who covers several techniques, for example a naturopath, who can draw up a programme of treatment to tackle each energy body. Individual therapies that focus on the immune system are those that affect the etheric body. Consider therapies from Classes 2, 3, 8, and 14.

▼
YES
▼

Your asthma is your body's way of complaining about being emotionally and mentally overwhelmed by your lifestyle.
Consider therapies that affect the emotional and mental bodies: Classes 3, 4, 5, 6, 10, 11, and 12. The more generalized Class 2 and 8 therapies are also useful.

▼
YES
▼

This may indicate an inherited weakness, likely to be in the etheric body.
Initially try a therapy from Class 2, 3, 8, or 14.

ORTHODOX TREATMENTS

Asthma is a potentially life-threatening condition, which orthodox medicine treats with bronchodilator and steroid drugs. These life-saving treatments are usually prescribed as inhalers, and taken regularly effectively suppress asthma symptoms. However they do not cure asthma, and they can cause side effects, trivial and serious.

These treatments provide invaluable support for asthma sufferers. While using energy-medicine techniques you should continue your prescribed medication, to support your body physically, until the energetic changes have activated your self-healing system.
● Do not stop your medication without first discussing this with your doctor.

4

Did your asthma follow a bad chest infection? ▸ NO ▸

YES

This is an immune system problem, likely to be in the etheric body.
Try therapies from Classes 2, 3, 8, or 14.

5

Do you have poor posture or back problems? ▸ NO

YES

Chronic asthma causes poor posture, making it more resistant to treatment because the chest cannot move normally.
To release the posture, try therapies from Classes 1, 4, or 6.

go to question 6 below

6

Did your asthma follow a major life stress (in the previous 9 months)? ▸ NO ▸

YES

Psychological difficulties in adjusting to your new lifestyle have led to difficulties in your immune system. This particularly affects your mental and emotional bodies, which influence the etheric body.
Try a Class 2, 3, 8, or 14 therapy for the etheric body. Also consider Class 5 and 6 therapies for the emotional body.
If you have recently moved house pay particular attention to Class 9 therapies, which affect the etheric body.
Your stress may be due to the way you perceive what has happened. Choose a Class 11 therapy that affects the mental body. To maintain equilibrium consider Class 4 or 12 disciplines.

7

Do you have difficulty expressing yourself emotionally? ▸ NO ▸

YES

Blockage of emotions often creates physical problems. You may not be conscious of this link, but this lack of awareness actually increases the asthma's emotional hold.
If you like working with your mind, try Class 11 techniques. If you find this hard or ineffective, consider Class 4, 7, or 10 techniques.

Your illness may be a sign that you need to make inner and outer changes in attitude and lifestyle. It is an indication that deep changes in consciousness are trying to take place. You will have to do most of the work from the inside, as it is a life problem that only you can resolve.
You may already have been disappointed by various therapies. The most useful are those that help you connect with your causal body, freeing up energy patterns in the other bodies. The therapies most able to do this are Classes 11 and 12, and also Classes 3, 4, 5, and 8. When you become stuck with an illness there may be an environmental cause. Consider Class 9 techniques.

CATARRH AND SINUS PROBLEMS

These problems can be or can become chronic and are hard to treat using both conventional or alternative treatments. Often a physical approach, such as dietary change, is beneficial, but this takes more discipline and time than many people are prepared to give for what is a relatively innocuous symptom.

①

Have you recently had an acute infection such as a cold or 'flu?

▸ NO ▸

▼
YES
▼

The catarrhal stage can last long after the virus has gone, as the mucous membranes have been unable to settle. This is probably due to physical causes. See box (p. 123) for physical methods to release the catarrh.
If physical causes cannot be detected or eliminated Class 2, 3, 8, or 14 techniques may help speed the process. They are able to access the etheric body, where the illness has become "stuck" and release it so that the normal pattern for health is resumed.

②

Are your symptoms worsened by dusty, mouldy, damp, or over-air-conditioned environments or possible allergens such as animal hair, chemicals, perfumes, or smoke?

▸ NO ▸

▼
YES
▼

Allergens set off an allergic reaction.
Try physical methods (see box, p. 123). In particular, drink plenty of water. If these methods fail or have limited effect, Class 2, 3, 8, or 14 techniques, which can stabilize the etheric body, may help.

③

Do you find it difficult to express your emotions, especially tears and grief? Or have you suffered a bereavement that you feel you might not have "got over"?

▸ NO ▸

▼
YES
▼

The catarrh may be due to repressed energy in the emotional body, which has become incorporated into a body symptom of blocked tears. Profuse tears mimic a catarrhal state, but once over the nose usually clears exceptionally well as the energy from the emotional body is released and no longer affects the etheric and physical bodies.
Therapies that encourage release of energies in the emotional body are: the psychotherapeutic techniques in Class 11; rebirthing and similar Class 7 techniques; and body-orientated techniques such as Class 5 active therapies and Class 6 passive therapies.

▸ NO ▸ ▸ ▸

ORTHODOX TREATMENTS

Orthodox treatment of catarrh is very poor. The use of nasal decongestants is rarely prescribed, as the nasal spray form aggravates the condition in the long term and tablets tend to be ineffective. If symptoms are due to an allergic response (allergic rhinitis) steroid-based nasal sprays or antihistamine tablets can be helpful.

4

▸ Did the catarrh follow a face or head injury?

YES

This may have disturbed the fine bony structure in the sinuses. *A Class 1 manipulation or Class 2 technique may be of use. These act on the physical body to stimulate the etheric body, where the trapped pattern is held.*

▸ **NO** ▸ **5**

Does this problem come and go?

YES

Stress, coupled with a mild degree of allergy, may combine to produce symptoms periodically. *Temporary improvement can be obtained by steam inhalation. Also Class 2, 3, 8, and 14 therapies are useful as long-term measures.*

▸ **NO** ▸ *If you cannot find a specific cause for your symptoms, it is likely that there is a mixture of causes. Some of the problem will be due to physical irritation, some due to an attempt by the body to release toxins, some due to physical distortions, and some may be of a psychosomatic nature.*
Look at dietary improvements and clean the environmental air that you breathe (see box below left). Therapies from Classes 2, 3, 8, and 14 can be used to help relieve this problem.
These include therapies that encourage drainage of toxins acting at the physical level; those that help to normalize the body's response to the environment at the etheric level; and also those that work at an emotional level to release trapped emotions.

Physical ways of releasing catarrh

The removal of mucus-forming foods from the diet, such as dairy, sugar, wheat (especially white flour), chocolate, and, in some people, orange and citrus may help. Goat and soya milk are less mucus-forming alternatives to dairy. See also Food sensitivities chart (p. 180).
Increase your fruit and vegetable intake – aim for 5 portions daily. A 48-hour water and pure juice fast is particularly effective. This helps toxin release.
Vitamins C and B complex in large doses also help catarrh and if there is infection involved echinacea is also good. Saline nasal washes and steam inhalation with aromatic oils, such as eucalyptus or cedar, also help, at least temporarily.

Reducing house dust (banning dust-carrying ornaments and furniture and using antidust pillow covers) can help reduce allergies. Air ionizers also help. Normalizing air temperature and humidity is also valuable. Reducing or changing medication (with your doctor's approval) may help catarrh when this seems to be related to starting a drug treatment.

● Catarrh is a very basic response to overload of the system with toxins. It often takes far longer to clear than one would expect, so that dietary or environmental changes may need to continue for months before any beneficial effects are noticed.

ECZEMA/1

1

a) Did your rash first appear at a young age (0–7 years)? ▶ NO ▶ ▶ ▶ ▶ ▶ ▶ ▶ ▶ ▶ ▶ ▶

YES
▼

b) Did either of your parents have asthma, eczema, or hayfever? ▶ NO ▶ *Go to question 3.*

YES
▼

Atopic illnesses are often inherited, implying that you have an innate tendency to a weakness in this area.
Treatments best suited to this level include Class 2 methods, particularly acupuncture combined with Chinese herbalism, and Class 8 or 14 techniques. These can all affect the etheric body, where much inherited illness has its main effect.

2

a) Has it started only recently? ▶ NO ▶ ▶ ▶

YES
▼

b) Does it affect only specific areas such as the hands, eyes, wrists, or navel? ▶ NO ▶ ▶ ▶

YES
▼

This may be contact dermatitis rather that classic eczema. Check clothing and jewellery for metal to which you may have developed an allergy. Also check cosmetics, soap powder (especially biological), and hair products, which can produce allergic reaction if you have used them for some time or have started them again after a break. *The best solution is to avoid the offending product. The rash may take a while to clear.*

▶ ▶ ▶ ▶ ▶ ▶ ▶ ▶ ▶ ▶ ▶ ▶ ▶

③

▶ Do you find that you easily become anxious or distressed?

▶NO▶ ④

▶ Do you find it difficult to express what you truly feel?

▶NO▶ go to next page

▼
YES
▼

▼
YES
▼

▶ ▶ If you feel there might be other factors contributing to your eczema, rejoin the chart at question 3.

The skin reacts strongly to stress and this can be a potent trigger for eczema. It is a subconscious reaction particularly affecting the emotional body.

Methods that help release emotional tensions can help to relieve skin problems. Psychotherapy techniques (Class 11) are useful, especially those that help in relaxation, such as hypnosis and autogenic training. Meditation (Class 12) is also a useful tool, as are Class 4 methods such as yoga and tai chi.

See ★ next page.

ORTHODOX TREATMENTS

The mainstay of orthodox treatment for eczema is the efficient use of moisturizers. This does not cure the condition, but makes the skin less prone to irritation. When this is not sufficient steroid-based creams or ointments are used. These can be dramatically effective, but prolonged use can damage and weaken the skin, making it even more liable to irritation. Occasionally people have to use steroids or other tablets that suppress the over-reactivity of the immune system that seems to underly eczema. Doctors recognize that eczema is aggravated by external irritants such as pet dander and house dust mites. Some put more emphasis on this than others. In practice some individuals find that these things are strong triggers, while others appear to be hardly affected.

ECZEMA/2

5

Are you easily irritated or do you easily feel ashamed?

▶ NO ▶

6

Have you moved house in the past 6 months?

▶ NO ▶

Your rash is perhaps an indicator that you need to look more deeply at your life and yourself. Your difficulties probably lie in your belief system, which is strongly affected by your emotions. This affects your mental and emotional bodies.

▼

YES

▼

★ Probably at an early age you developed a fear of truly expressing feelings. You may remember incidents that made you feel this way. These fears disturb the emotional body and create false beliefs in the mental body.

Therapies which can free up the emotional energy and allow beliefs to change can be useful. Class 5 movement therapies and Class 11 psychotherapies can help free your emotional expression. The effects can filter down to the physical body and help relieve the eczema.

▼

YES

▼

You may be allergic to something in the house, particularly animal dander, mould, or house mites. Wash or replace old furnishings, and deal with damp.

If physical factors are not a problem you may be picking up the effects of environmental stress. If others around you notice that they are more prone to illness or psychological upset, environmental stress is a likely cause.

See Class 9 methods, which deal with these effects on the subtle bodies.

Consider a psychological technique (Class 11). Classes 4, 5, 6, 8, and 14 all complement this approach and can be used independently. Classes 3 and 12 are good to link you directly to your causal body – this in itself overcomes the need for much illness.

Food allergy and eczema

Many people are aware that eczema is an allergic reaction. This has generated much interest in dietary allergens in eczema. Complementary medicine generally supports the idea that diet is a major factor in the development of eczema, but orthodox doctors are unconvinced that this is true for the majority of sufferers. If you suspect that your eczema may have a food allergy component, see the Food sensitivities chart (p.180).

RECURRENT VIRAL INFECTIONS/1

1

a) Is the sufferer a child under 12 years of age? ▶ NO ▶

go to next page

▼
YES
▼

Check with your doctor to make sure that there is no underlying illness that might be making the child more prone to infection. This is a rare possibility, but should be considered. (Once this is excluded continue the chart.)

▼
YES
▼

b) Does the child seem to recover slowly and/or does s/he regularly develop complications such as earache?

▶ NO ▶ c) Has the child, or have any siblings, recently started, or moved, school?

▶ NO ▶ Some children are simply more prone to viral illnesses. Try the support measures given in the box (p. 128). If these do not work the child may not be suffering from viral infections but from a food intolerance, which can either mimic an infection or else make the child more prone to infections.
To discover whether this might be a problem see the Food sensitivities chart (p. 180).

▼
YES
▼

This suggests that the immune system is struggling. The problem is likely to be at the etheric level, where the impact of infections first registers.
Classes 8 and 14 can strengthen the immune system. Class 2 therapies are also helpful, but they are less child-friendly.

▼
YES
▼

This exposes a child to a whole new range of viruses that s/he may not have had contact with before. Catching and dealing with infections is part of the way the immune system develops.
Try the support measures given in the box (p. 128). These help the physical body develop the immune system.

ORTHODOX TREATMENTS

Recent research shows that most recurrent infections are caused by viruses for which there is no drug treatment. The use of antibiotics to treat viruses is useless (antibiotics attack bacteria and have no effect on viruses). Inappropriate use of antibiotics increases bacterial resistance, which can make treatment of serious bacterial illnesses difficult, especially in those with poor natural defences. Also antibiotics change gut flora, leaving one vulnerable to food intolerance (see p. 180). Treatment of viral infections is simply a matter of relieving pains and fever with aspirin, paracetamol, or over-the-counter medicines containing these, and drinking plenty of fluid.

RECURRENT VIRAL INFECTIONS/2

2

Does your work involve high stress levels (e.g. deadlines, overtime, weekend work, night work, travel and overnight stays, or a high level of socializing, with rich food and drink)?

▼
YES
▼

The mind can cope with, and even enjoy, stress. But if physical and emotional needs are constantly over-ridden, health may suffer. Stress lowers the effectiveness of the immune system, so you may need to reassess your lifestyle.
Therapies to help you relax and use free time better include Class 1 aromatherapy and massage, and Class 2 shiatsu and reflexology. Classes 3, 4, 5, 6, 7, 11, and 12 all help in various ways. These therapies can affect all the subtle bodies, but the effect on the emotional body is particularly helpful. Choose a therapy which is enjoyable and nurturing.

▸ NO ▸

3

Do you work in any of the following environments: a school, a medical establishment, an institution, a crowded office with air-conditioning?

▼
YES
▼

All these environments expose you to a higher level of viruses than normal. Make sure you physically support your body (see Support measures box, below). Also continue the chart. You may have other factors that are contributing to your low resistance to infection.

▸ NO ▸

4

Has your susceptibility to infections started since a bereavement or a similar traumatic emotional event?

▼
YES
▼

Such emotional traumas lower the effectiveness of the immune system. The emotional body is disturbed by the shock.
Therapies that work with the emotional body are useful. Class 3 therapies also connect you to your causal body, which is especially valuable when you have experienced a loss. Class 7 and 12 therapies are also useful in this way. Psychological therapies (Class 11) are also helpful to encourage the processing of emotions that are necessary to restore equilibrium to the emotional body.

▸ NO ▸ ▸ ▸

Support measures

Certain vitamins, minerals, and herbs are thought to help prevent or treat these kinds of infection. Medical research has been interested in these less orthodox treatments, but as yet no clear evidence has proved their effectiveness. Vitamin C in high doses spread through the day has a good reputation and smaller doses can help prevention. Zinc lozenges are also useful as a treatment, but need to be taken frequently. For post-infection lethargy high doses of B complex for one month can be useful. Echinacea is also a well-tried treatment. Resting, drinking plenty of water, and avoiding dairy products and sweets can aid recovery from viral infection. These treatments act at a physical level.

5

▶ ▶ Do you fail to eat a mostly wholefood-type diet, with at least 5 portions of fruit and vegetables daily?

▶ **NO** ▶

▼

YES

▼

A high-sugar, high-fat, high-protein diet, low in fruit and vegetables, stresses the body physically, making it more prone to infections.
Try adjusting your diet and following the advice in the Support measures box (p.128).

6

Do you lack an active and enjoyable social life?

▶ **NO** ▶

▼

YES

▼

This makes you more prone to infections, possibly because your emotional body is unfulfilled. Try improving your social life.
Therapies which may help are Classes 4, 5, and 7, which improve energy flow in your emotional body, in turn improving your resistance. They also provide social contact.

7

Have you started to get more frequent infections since moving house?

▶ **NO** ▼

▼

YES

▼

Assuming that there are no physical factors (e.g. air-conditioning, over- or under-heating, or damp) making you more prone to illness, you may be suffering from the effect of adverse energies in your home.
See Class 9 therapies such as the treatment of geopathic stress.

go to question 8 below

▼
▼
▼
▼
▼
▼
▼
▼
▼
▼
▼
▼
▼

◀ ◀

▼

8

Do you keep getting low-grade, viral-type illnesses that never really turn into a proper "cold" or which go on for a prolonged time?

▼

YES

▼

You may have a food intolerance. See the Food sensitivities chart on p. 180.

▶ **NO** ▶ *If you have still not found a cause and there is no medical cause, perhaps an inner change in consciousness is trying to take place – possibly the need to contact your causal body. You may need to change your belief system relating to your mental body or to your emotional responses that affect your emotional body. Changes can filter through to the physical and so boost the immune system. Therapies most able to help include Classes 3, 7, 11, and 12. Others, which have a more general effect on the etheric body, include Classes 2, 8, and 14.*

ANXIETY/1

Anxiety is a psychological and physical state, experienced as worry, forgetfulness, insecurity, loss of confidence, sleeplessness, inability to relax, irritability, or irrepressible fears. Physically it can also produce light-headedness, headaches, disturbance of appetite, digestive and bowel upsets, chest pains, shortness of breath, and palpitations. Physical symptoms of anxiety can be the same as those caused by other illnesses, so see your doctor before consulting this chart.

1

Are you between 9 and 18 years of age? ▸ **NO** ▸

▼
YES
▼

This period of adolescence is when anxiety may be stimulated by growth, hormonal, and social changes. This is a time of transition, and it occurs in your mental, emotional, and etheric bodies as well as your physical body.
Therapies affecting all the subtle bodies are useful. Consider Class 3, 7, and 8 therapies. Also look at taking up, as a long-term discipline, a Class 4 or 12 therapy. If your problems are mainly psychological consider a Class 11 therapy.

2

Are you a woman and do you have spells of anxiety at the same time in your menstrual cycle? ▸ **NO** ▸

▼
YES
▼

Your anxiety is likely to be a symptom of PMS.
See the PMS chart (p.159).

3

Have you recently become pregnant or given birth? ▸ **NO** ▸ ▸ ▸

▼
YES
▼

In pregnancy, changes in hormone levels affect the etheric body. You may not be adjusting well to these changes.
Consider a Class 2, 8, or 14 therapy to help you adapt. You may also be experiencing apprehension about your new role in life. This affects your mental and emotional bodies. If you feel this is an important aspect also consider Class 3 or 11 therapies, which will help the emotional and mental bodies.

ORTHODOX TREATMENTS

Anxiety is treated with the same drugs as those used to treat depression, since depression often underlies the anxiety.

The use of anti-anxiety drugs such as the benzodiazepines (e.g. Valium) is now avoided, except for one-off stresses such as fear of flying. This is because these drugs have been found to be addictive. If anxiety is mainly producing physical symptoms Beta blockers (used in lower doses for high blood pressure and heart disease) can be helpful.

Even when orthodox treatment is used, psychotherapy of some sort is often beneficial.

4

▶ Are you a woman of perimenopausal age (38 years or older) and do you have some menopausal symptoms such as hot flushes, changes in your menstrual cycle, aches and pains, memory loss, or poor sleep?

▼
YES
▼

The changes of the menopause are occurring in your physical and etheric bodies.
Your anxiety is likely to be part of your menopausal process.
Refer to the Menopause chart (see p.167).

5

▶ NO ▶ Are you having a new life experience that should be exciting and fun, such as a new baby or a relationship?

▼
YES
▼

The situation is too much for your emotional body, probably because of some of your mental attitudes. What should be felt as excitement is upsetting you.
Consider therapies that help the emotional and mental bodies, such as Classes 3, 7, 8, and 11.

6

▶ NO ▶ Do you become anxious when anticipating a worrying event, such as an exam, a flight, or an interview?

▼
YES
▼

This situation is too much for your emotional body, probably because of your mental beliefs.
As a first-aid measure consider a Class 2, 8, or 11 therapy. Other therapies that affect the emotional and mental bodies, such as Class 3, may also be useful. If you always have an underlying state of anxiety, consider regularly practising a Class 4 or 12 technique. A Class 13 technique will also help you keep a quiet centre.

▶ NO ▶

go to next page

ANXIETY/2

7

Are you experiencing insecurity from loss of health, job, or income, of a loved one, or of your role in your family or community?

▶ NO ▶

▼
YES
▼

The anxiety may have been triggered by the realization that nothing can be relied upon to be permanent, destroying a commonly held belief system in the mental body. Your emotional body is responding to this by feeling fear and grief. This state is a strong place to grow from.
See general advice box, below.

8

Do you find yourself worrying about unlikely but awful things that might happen, such as developing cancer or your child being run over?

▶ NO ▶

▼
YES
▼

This kind of thought pattern comes from not being in touch with your causal body. You have allowed your belief system to be based on externals, leading to distortions of perception. For example, constantly watching news and disaster films has impressed on you that this is normal reality. Your belief system has to detach and reconnect to your causal self, to give you support or guidance.
See general advice box, below.

9

Do you rarely get time for yourself?

▶ NO ▶   ▶   ▶

▼
YES
▼

This may either be the cause or the effect of your anxiety. Lack of space and time for relaxation and reflection prevents you from contacting your causal body, and this is anxiety-producing. Or you may be resisting opening up this contact out of fear of what might be revealed – you have filled up your life with so much that contact is avoided. In either case the anxiety will be relieved if the contact is encouraged.
See general advice box, below.
It is particularly important for you to find a regular time to practise a Class 4 or 12 technique, to help build up contact with the causal body.

General advice

Therapies that can help you to adjust your belief system (and hence affect the mental body) and reconnect you with your causal body can be helpful. Consider Class 8 and 11 therapies to help the mental body and Class 3, 7, and 12 to help the causal body connection. However, all therapies have the possibility of helping you reconnect to this level.

⑩

▶ ▶ Are you unable to express yourself physically and emotionally as you would like to? ▶ **NO** ▶

▼
YES
▼

This curbing of expression affects your emotional body and generates a tension that you experience as anxiety. The problem probably originated in the mental body as beliefs that you cannot or should not freely express yourself.
Consider Class 5, 6, 7, 8, and 11 therapies, which will help you free up your ways of expression.

⑪

Do you get a lot of vague physical symptoms, such as light-headedness, headaches, feeling unreal, poor memory or concentration, as well as anxiety? ▶ **NO** ▶

▼
YES
▼

You may be generating anxiety by the way you breathe. You may be hyperventilating – breathing too shallowly so that levels of carbon dioxide in your blood are too low. This alters the metabolism in the brain, causing vague physical symptoms and anxiety. Learning how to breathe using the diaphragm may greatly relieve symptoms.
Also consider trying a Class 4, 7, or 11 therapy, which can help you to relax and breathe properly.

⑫

Do you have an unavoidable, constant level of tension in your life, such as chronic illness, money worries, or a difficult relationship? ▶ **NO** ▼

▼
YES
▼

There are two ways to deal with this type of anxiety. The first is to see if something can be changed in your life. The other is to become more impervious to the problem. Once detachment is achieved an attainable solution to the stress may appear.
This can be achieved by altering your beliefs – a Class 11 therapy can be helpful. But the most fundamental way is to re-establish contact with your causal body. This sees beyond material and emotional problems and is in touch with peace and contentment. Class 3, 8, and 12 therapies can help.

go to question 13 below

◀ ◀

▼

⑬

Do you have a constant undercurrent of anxiety throughout your life, whatever is going on? ▶ **NO** ▶

▼
YES
▼

This is probably due to being out of touch with your causal body. You cannot achieve true peace if you are unaware of who you really are and your purpose in life.
See general advice box (p. 132).

If you are unable to find a cause for your anxiety from this chart, see your doctor, as you may have a physical condition, such as hyperthyroidism, which generates the symptoms of anxiety.

HYPERTENSION

1

Do you have other health problems that affect the cardiovascular system such as angina, a stroke, diabetes, raised cholesterol, or heart failure, **or** do any of these conditions run in your family, **or** do you have kidney problems?

▶ NO ▶

▼
YES
▼

In your case it is particularly important that high blood pressure is well controlled – if it continues to remain high your risk of developing worse symptoms is increased. If you are going to try energy healing you will need the support of your doctor. You may need to continue some of your drugs, and you should not stop them abruptly. Your illness is affecting your physical body as well as your subtle bodies.

Therapies that are the most help are those which treat several levels of the subtle bodies. Consider Class 2, 8, or 14 therapies. Also rejoin the chart to see if there are other factors that may influence your blood pressure.

2

Are you overweight?

▶ NO ▶

▼
YES
▼

Weight plays a significant role in raising blood pressure. Simply reducing your weight may bring your blood pressure within normal limits. You will also gain health benefits by stopping smoking and increasing exercise. These methods all act primarily on the physical body, but the sense of wellbeing will affect the etheric and even the emotional body. For energy-healing suggestions continue with the chart.

3

Do you find yourself constantly in a rush or pushed to meet deadlines?

▶ NO ▶ ▶ ▶

▼
YES
▼

You are constantly asking your body to operate in overdrive. This overstimulates the adrenals, releasing hormones that affect blood pressure. Eventually the rise in blood pressure will become chronic.
See Coping with stress box, below.

Coping with stress

The pattern of constantly creating and living in stress is a powerful incubator of ill health, such as hypertension. The solution is not necessarily to remove stress but to learn to cope with it. This means learning to relax, enjoying relaxation, and learning new ways of moving through stress-provoking situations.

Consider Class 1 massage or aromatherapy, which affect the physical, etheric, and emotional bodies, to relieve tensions held in the being. Class 2 therapies help in a similar way. Class 4 disciplines are relaxing and can alter your attitude to dealing with stress by introducing new ways of being in your body.

Class 11 therapies, especially autogenic training and hypnosis, have a similar effect to Class 4 disciplines, but by altering mental and emotional attitudes (and bodies). Meditation (Class 12) is useful in this way, too, and also connects you to your causal body. A deeper connection to this is a profound reliever of stress. Class 3 therapies also help.

Do you find you have no time for yourself?

▼

YES

▼

Make time for yourself a priority. Without this you are in a constant "putting-out" cycle, which eventually becomes stress you cannot release.
See Coping with stress box (p.134).

▶ NO ▶ Do you find it difficult to relax?

▼

YES

▼

This is something you need to learn to do consciously. Many energy-healing methods use relaxation as the first step in the healing process.
See Coping with stress box (p.134).

▶ NO ▶ Do you find you are easily provoked to anger or tears?

▼

YES

▼

You are being too easily triggered into a stress-provoking emotional reaction.
Class 11 therapies, which work on the mental and emotional bodies, help you to see situations in a new and less stressful way.
See also the Coping with stress box (p.134).

▶ NO ▼

go to question 7 below

◀ ◀

▼

7 Do you find it difficult to express emotion?

▼

YES

▼

This build-up of energy in the emotional body is highly disturbing to the integrated functioning of the subtle bodies.
See Coping with stress box (p.134).

▶ NO ▶ Raised blood pressure is unusual as it is not normally accompanied by symptoms. It is the long-term effects that it may trigger that are the concern. It may be that your blood pressure is right for you. However, statistically people with lower blood pressure are better protected against cardiovascular disease. To help reduce your blood pressure and also improve overall health an energy-healing method can help – especially if the reading is borderline.
Consider a Class 2, 8, or 14 therapy, which has an holistic effect on your subtle bodies and can help to bring your physical and subtle bodies into an alignment that is free of disease.

Limitations of drugs

Recent studies have shown that even with medically treated hypertension, there is an increased likelihood of cardiovascular illness compared with a naturally normal blood pressure. This indicates that it is not just the raised blood pressure that is the problem. Lowering your blood pressure using an energy-based method brings it to a normal level in a natural way, which should also eliminate the other, as yet unknown, disease-provoking factors that go along with raised blood pressure. These treatments act outward from the subtle to the physical levels, while orthodox drugs only act on the blood pressure component of the condition.

DEPRESSION/1

❶

Have you experienced loss recently – a bereavement (including pets), or the breakup of a relationship?

▼
YES
▼

Your depression is probably tied in with the grieving process. All these events tend to trigger a grief reaction as a response to loss. A major loss affects all the subtle bodies, but especially the emotional body.
See Dealing with grief box, below.

▸ **NO** ▸

❷

Have you recently experienced a major lifestyle change, such as children leaving home, loss of earnings, loss of job or retirement, or leaving home?

▼
YES
▼

This is a kind of bereavement. The process of the resolution of grief occurs when the mental body has been able to adjust to the new reality. This allows the emotional body to return to normal.
See Dealing with grief box, below.

▸ **NO** ▸

❸

a) Has your family recently been extended by a new baby?

▼
YES
▼

b) Are you the mother?

▼
YES
▼

You may be suffering from post-natal depression, which is mainly due to sudden changes in female hormones after birth. A feeling of anti-climax and the strain of disturbed nights may be adding to the problem. Discuss your feelings with your doctor or midwife. You may need orthodox medical attention.
To help your physical body adjust, eat well and avoid convenience foods and sweet snacks. Eat plenty of fresh fruit and vegetables and wholegrain cereals.
Hormonal changes will have disturbed your etheric and physical bodies.
A Class 2, 8, or 14 therapy will help to readjust this, as these act primarily on the etheric body. If these methods do not help, continue with the chart.

▸ **NO** ▸ ▸ ▸ ▸

▸ **NO** ▸ ▸ ▸ ▸

Dealing with grief

Overcoming grief is a natural process. However, it can become "stuck". Many alternative therapies can help to free up the process. Therapies that concentrate on the mental body, such as Class 11 therapies, or therapies that affect all the subtle bodies and help connection to the causal body (such as Classes 3 and 12), are very helpful.

Class 8 therapies, particularly Bach flower remedies, are also useful. If there are mixed or unexpressed emotions, common in grief reactions, therapies that help the emotional body, such as Class 5, 6, and 7 therapies, are also to be considered. These help to free up the emotional body.

go to next page

▶ ▶

4

Have you noticed that your depression comes on in the autumn and lifts in the spring?

▶ **NO** ▶

▼

YES

▼

You may be suffering from seasonal affective disorder (SAD) – the depression triggered by the short daylight hours of winter. Or you may simply get "winter blues", suggesting that your inner wellbeing is overly affected by external changes, affecting your emotional body.

Try full-spectrum lighting for work areas or a therapeutic full-spectrum light box. Also look at your lifestyle. Lack of exercise and an unhealthy diet high in sugars and fat and low in fruit and vegetables makes it hard for your body to generate feelings of wellbeing.

Finally, you need to find "inner light", which can be done by looking at your belief systems (or mental body) and your emotional expression (emotional body). *Changes in belief systems can be helped by Class 8 and 11 therapies. These can also help your emotional expression, as can Classes 5 and 7. Class 3 and 12 therapies, which help access the causal body, are also useful.*

▶ ▶ You may be feeling grief at the loss of the old life, plus the effects of stress that a new baby can produce. This may be further aggravated if you expected acceptance and joy. Not being able to accept or express feelings fully may make you bottle them up, resulting in depression. Your mental and emotional bodies are affected.

Therapies that concentrate on the mental and the emotional bodies may be helpful, for example a Class 11 psychotherapy, a Class 5 dance therapy, or a Class 7 breathing therapy. Class 8 therapies, primarily affecting the etheric body, may also be useful. It is important to share feelings with your family so that you can give each other emotional and practical support.

DEPRESSION/2

5

Are you living under the stress of an unsatisfactory relationship (not necessarily with your partner), money, work, or housing worries? ▶ NO ▶

▼
YES
▼

Your emotional body is unable to respond freely to these pressures and shuts down. This is the feeling of depression. Seek counselling, as you may be overlooking good solutions. You may also need to face up to reality and take courage to make major changes. External support is useful. If you sort out practical problems your depression may lift, as the emotional body is no longer stressed. *If not, look at ways of changing your belief system (mental body), for example, by using a Class 11 therapy or by opening up to the causal body. These can help transform a good situation from a bad one. Class 3 therapies are good for this. The other approach is to help your emotional body free itself. Class 5, 6, or 8 therapies are good for this. To relieve the stress on the whole of your system a Class 4 technique, such as tai chi or yoga, would be a beneficial long-term therapy.*

6

Have you noticed that you suffer from an inexplicable or easily triggered depression, or do you get periods of "highs" and "lows"? ▶ NO ▶

▼
YES
▼

You may be suffering from, bipolar affective disorder (BAD). This may need orthodox medical treatment – see your doctor before continuing this chart. Some people have a variable emotional life that is not as extreme as BAD. If so you would benefit from having better control of emotional responses. *Therapies that improve contact with your causal body are very useful, as this body experiences what lies beyond everyday ups and downs. Class 3 or 7 therapies are useful. Contact can also be accessed via the physical body by practising Class 4 techniques, which work on all the energy bodies. Class 12 techniques also help contact the causal body and stabilize mental and emotional bodies. If you feel your problem is aggravated by emotions never being freely expressed, try a Class 5, 6, or 11 technique to free up the emotional body.*

7

a) Do you regularly drink more than 21 units of alcohol a week? ▶ NO ▶ ▶ ▶

▼
YES
▼

b) Would you answer "yes" to 2 or more of these questions: ▶ NO ▶ ▶ ▶
● Are you ever concerned about the amount you drink?
● Are people around you concerned about the amount you drink?
● Have you ever missed work or been late as a result of drinking?
● Do you ever feel guilty about your drinking?

▼
YES
▼

You may be suffering from alcoholism. See the Addiction chart (p.141), as well as continuing with this chart.

8

▶ ▶ a) Do you use recreational drugs, such as cannabis, most days?

▶ **NO** ▶ ▶ ▶ ▶ ▶ ▶ ▶ ▶ ▶ ▶ ▶

▼
YES
▼

▶ ▶ b) Were you having problems with moods before you started taking alcohol or drugs ?

▶ **NO** ▶ One of the side effects of alcohol or drugs is depression. Stop taking them.
See the Addiction chart (p.141). This should restore normal mood patterns, though it may take some time.

▼
YES
▼

You may have started using drugs or alcohol as a way of "self-medicating" depression. This often happens subconsciously, as in the initial stages they do improve mood. Over time this effect may be reversed, adding to your depression rather than relieving it.
Stop taking these substances and see your doctor, as you may need professional help. Also see the Addiction chart (p.141). If you want to supplement this with a complementary therapy, rejoin this chart.

9

▶ Are you drawn to philosophical, religious, or spiritual interests, or do you feel depressed about the state of humankind?

▶ **NO** ▶

go to next page

▼
YES
▼

This type of mental interest often leads to depression. The mental body is being overused. This may be an attempt to numb the emotional body because it has been hurt. To overcome this both the causal and the emotional body need to be opened up. For someone stuck in a "mind space" physical or emotionally based therapies are good – but are often avoided.
Therapies such as those in Class 3 that access all the subtle bodies, Class 5, 6, and 8, which access the emotional body, or Class 4 therapies, which are physical but open up all the subtle bodies, are useful. Class 11 therapies are also helpful, but you need to make sure you break through your pattern of intellectualizing your problems. I would discourage meditation, though it does open up the causal body, as it is not physical or emotional enough and can aggravate the problem.

DEPRESSION/3

⑩

Are you suffering from a chronic illness?

▸ NO ▸

▼

YES

▼

Physical illness undermines well-being. If this becomes chronic, not only do you have to deal with the illness but also the mental and emotional effects of having to endure chronic disabilities, limitation of freedom, and fears about the future, which can manifest as depression.
Class 3 therapies, which tend to focus on the healthy rather than the ill parts of the body and also connect all our bodies to the causal body, are beneficial.
Class 2 and 8 therapies, which may also have an overall beneficial effect on the disease, are useful. These affect the etheric body, but the other subtle bodies are also accessed. The disciplines of Class 4 are also useful in a similar way.
Class 5, 6, and 7 therapies are especially useful to free up the emotional body, which is particularly affected by the depression of chronic illness. Maximizing the healing effects of your environ-ment may also help. Consider a Class 9 or 10 technique.

⑪

Does your depression relate to certain buildings or rooms, for example does it come on after being in certain places?

▸ NO ▸

▼

YES

▼

You may be sensitive to the energy of the environment and this is affecting your subtle bodies – particularly your emotional body, which is closing down to protect itself, leaving you feeling depressed.
If it is your own home, consider a Class 9, 10, or a Class 11 technique. These should clear or neutralize energies affecting you. If it is triggered away from home, a power object may help (see p.111). Class 3 therapies that strengthen your connection to your causal self are also useful.

If you have come to the end of this chart without identifying a cause, see your doctor again. Some physical illnesses, such as hypothyroidism or anaemia, can produce depression.
If a physical condition is not the cause of your depression this may indicate that you need to look more deeply at your life and yourself. Your difficulty probably lies in your belief system, which has affected your emotional body, producing the depression.
Consider a psychological technique such as a Class 11 therapy. Class 3, 4, 5, and 7 therapies all work well in conjunction with these as they either free up the emotional body (Classes 5 and 7) or help integrate all the subtle bodies (Classes 3 and 4).

ORTHODOX TREATMENTS

Depression is treated primarily with antidepressants. These drugs are not supposed to be addictive and aim to restore the brain's "natural" happiness-producing chemicals, such as serotonin. They take a month to get into the system fully and need to be taken at an effective dosage in order for the maximum benefit to be gained. These drugs are often used in combination with psychotherapy or counselling. They may have side effects such as a dry mouth, constipation, or blurred vision. However, the side effects tend to diminish with time and, if the drug works, are a minor irritation compared with the symptoms of depression. They can be used in conjunction with energy medicine.

ADDICTION/1

Addiction is a behaviour pattern that is difficult to resist. An addiction tends to mould your lifestyle to fit its needs rather than vice versa. Addictions are common with certain drugs, such as heroin, but nicotine, alcohol, and caffeine are also addictive.

Some people find certain foods addictive, while others become addicted to activities such as gambling, sex, exercise, shopping, or work, which seems to give them a "high". Some people tend more toward addiction than others.

1 Is your addiction to food, such as chocolate or sweets? ▶ NO ▶

▼
YES
▼

See the Eating disorders chart (p.170)

2 Are you addicted to a drug that was originally prescribed medically? ▶ NO ▶

▼
YES
▼

See your doctor. Some drugs, such as benzodiazepines (e.g. Valium) are hard to withdraw from and you will need medical help. For some medications there may be non-addictive alternatives. If not then it is better not to worry about addiction if the drugs are generally helpful. If you no longer want to take the drug and do not have an addictive nature then diet, acupuncture, and hypnosis (see box below) should give enough support to stop the medication.
If you have an addictive nature continue the chart.

3 Have you noticed that when you abstain from your addiction you start to feel unwell physically, and when you restart it you feel "right" again? ▶ NO ▶

▼
YES
▼

This indicates that you have a physical addiction to the substance or behaviour (such as "runner's high"). This is common and unexpectedly persistent with some substances, such as caffeine and nicotine. Your physical and etheric body has adapted to the addiction. The boxes on ear acupuncture (p. 145), hypnosis (below left), and diet (p. 142) will help you overcome this level of the addiction.
Try these before continuing with the chart. They will free up the energy in your etheric body, so that you will notice the benefits of changes occurring at more subtle levels.

go to next page

Hypnosis

Hypnosis can be used to help break addiction, having the advantage over other psychological methods in that it passes directly to the subconscious. However most addictions are held in place by more than the habit. During the session the hypnotist will help you access your subconscious to see if you are able and willing, at a deep level, to break the habit. If not, you are likely to need to do more work with subconscious patterns before the addiction habit can be released.

ADDICTION/2

4

Do you tend to be impatient, do you want your needs met instantly, or do you find yourself easily frustrated and disillusioned?

▸ NO ▸

▼
YES
▼

This is typical addict-type behaviour. Modifying it is a major step to recovery. Following advice in the boxes on diet (below right), ear acupuncture (p. 145), and hypnosis (p. 141) will help stabilize the physical and etheric bodies and make you less prone to these feelings.
Next, learning a discipline such as a Class 4 technique can help stabilize energy in all your subtle bodies. Alternatively try a Class 5 method, enabling you to connect with your emotional body directly, allowing you to express yourself more clearly. Class 11 psychological techniques can also help self-expression and understanding of one's being, so that impulsive behaviour is understood and new outlets are discovered. This works on the emotional and mental bodies. Rejoin this chart if you need more information.

5

Is your life highly stressful?

▸ NO ▸

▼
YES
▼

See ★ right.

6

Were you prone to anxiety or depression before the addiction became a problem?

▸ NO ▸

▼
YES
▼

★ Addictions disturb energy flow in the emotional body, making it less vulnerable to outside situations. This gives temporary relief. However addictions also damage the etheric and physical body, resulting in physical illness. *Choose a technique to stabilize the emotional body and reinforce the connection to your causal body. Consider Class 3, 4, 5, 7, 11, and 12 techniques.*

▸ NO ▸ ▸ ▸

Diet and addictions

It is common for an addict to substitute one addictive substance for another that is "less harmful". For example, alcoholics move to caffeine and sugary foods, heroin addicts move to cannabis. This removes the person to a less harmful situation, but does little to deal with the addictive tendency. For some this is satisfactory, but for others life becomes a struggle against resisting the temptation to relapse and they cannot open up to new experiences to replace the addiction.

Abstinence from alcohol has been shown to be much more successfully maintained if alcoholics eat a wholefood, caffeine- and sugar-free diet, with plenty of raw fruit and vegetables. This diet has been shown to reduce impulsive behaviour

markedly — part of the addictive pattern. The change in diet makes it easier for the addict to abstain, although initially changing both the addiction pattern and diet habits may seem overwhelming. The dietary change can probably be relaxed after 6 to 9 months.

Such a diet in part helps to replace any trace nutrients lacking which can make addictive tendencies worse. Also the diet stabilizes blood sugar levels; fluctuations in blood sugar can lead to emotional instability and compulsive tendencies.

On a subtle body level the physical and etheric bodies become more stable, so that changes for the better in the emotional and mental body, as well as the physical, are noticeable sooner.

Do you lack confidence or feel insecure, or do you seem confident and secure, when deep down you know this to be a facade?

▼
YES
▼

Addictive behaviour and drugs can give a false sense of importance, security, and success. They allow the emotional body to create feelings based on illusion. When you try to break an addiction, true feelings of aloneness, vulnerability, and lack of confidence resurface. This commonly causes people to relapse. To overcome this distortion in the emotional body, find new ways of seeing and patterns of behaviour.
Class 11 techniques can be very useful here. Other techniques to support this process are Class 3, 4, 5, 7, and 12. These all help to free the emotional body and increase connectedness to the causal body.

▶NO▶

Do you have difficulties with your close relationships?

▼
YES
▼

An addict's primary relationship is with his or her addiction. With this illusionary relationship in place it becomes difficult, if not impossible, to connect with others at the level of the subtle bodies. It is subtle body connection that leads to close and satisfying relationships.
See Spirituality and addiction box, below.

▶NO▶

9

Do you find it hard to participate fully in life – such as making friends and pursuing hobbies?

▼
YES
▼

See ★ p.144.

▶NO▶

see the spirituality and addiction box, below, and then go to next page

---

Spirituality and addiction

Deeply held addiction, especially to alcohol and drugs, is particularly hard to overcome. The most successful approach, which has to be followed by addicts themselves, is that of aligning to a source of spirituality. This is the approach of the well-known 12-step programme, devised by Alcoholics Anonymous. In this programme, whatever an addict recognizes as "God" becomes a focus for a new way of living. Many addicts have an innate understanding of the spiritual or energetic dimensions of life. It may be over-sensitivity in this area that triggered the need for chemical addiction initially, as mind-altering chemicals affect the subtle bodies, especially the emotional and mental. They become more rigid and impermeable to subtle energies. This acts as a protection mechanism. Part of the process of recovery is becoming able to protect the subtle bodies without the need for drugs or alcohol. Aligning to one's own "God" is a powerful way of achieving this. If the addiction to chemicals can be overcome, recovering addicts are often able to bring spirituality and awareness of subtle energies into everyday life. This gives them the ability to provide wisdom and healing of exceptional quality.

ADDICTION/3

⑩

Do you feel that no-one understands or cares about you?

▶NO▶

▼

YES

▼

★ Most addictions, especially drugs and alcohol, create bonhomie and connectedness to everything. These are illusionary and paradoxically can make you unavailable at the emotional level. As a result it is harder for you to connect with your life and relationships. This is because of the distortion of energy in the emotional body that addictions cause.

Therapies working with the emotional body to integrate it with the other subtle bodies can help break this pattern. Those that also connect you to your causal body are especially useful (see the Spirituality and addiction box, p.143). Class 3, 5, 7, 11, and 12 techniques might be helpful.

⑪

Do you feel that a "straight" life is dull, boring, or pointless?

▶NO▶

▼

YES

▼

Your life may be dull or boring, but how you live is influenced by your desire. If this has become channelled into addiction, life will seem pointless. The "highs", produced by an addictive habit, are part of the natural range of emotional life and can be achieved without addiction. Part of recovery is to learn to experience good feelings without addiction. Set yourself new creative and emotionally rewarding goals. Establishing a good connection with your causal body is important.

Class 3, 7, 11, and 12 techniques can be helpful. Try to view your life in a new and positive way. Class 5 therapies can help to free up your emotional expression. All these methods free up the energy of the emotional body, re-establish the conscious connection with the causal body, and re-align the energy of all the subtle bodies. See also the Spirituality and addiction box (p.143).

⑫

Do you, or did you as a child, feel over-sensitive to "atmosphere" or to the feelings of others, or did you have "psychic" abilities?

▶NO▶ ▶ ▶

▼

YES

▼

Addictions block the energies moving in the emotional body. People who are naturally over-sensitive or super-sensitive may use this unconsciously to block out over-intense messages. To release your addiction you need to learn to protect your emotional body. One of the best ways is to establish a more conscious connection to your causal body (see Spirituality and addiction box, p.143).

Class 3 methods are good to develop this connection and they help re-acquaint you with the experiences of subtle energies you are likely to have naturally. Class 4 methods are similarly useful. You may also consider Class 9 environmental treatments and Class 13 talismans and crystals. (Meditation, Class 12, is also useful.) These methods are all ways to protect you from your environment and the energies of others. You may find that you want to develop your gifts by becoming acquainted with a therapy – a good first step.

⓭

▶ ▶ Do you need to break your addiction because it is damaging your health? ▶ NO ▶

▼

YES

▼

It is likely that the addiction is not having such a distorting effect on your emotional body, but it is affecting your etheric and causal bodies, which is just as devastating.
The guidlines on diet (p.142), or ear acupuncture (below), and hypnosis (p.141) should help by supporting the physical and etheric bodies and allowing any blocks at the emotional level to surface and be dealt with.

⓮

Do you wish to break from the addiction because you believe, or have been led to believe, that it is bad for you? ▶ NO ▶

▼

YES

▼

If you have come to the end of this chart without gaining insight into the nature of your addictive process, it is likely that your physical and subtle bodies are not being disturbed much by the addiction. However if you wish to break your habit the guidelines on diet (p.142), ear acupuncture (below), and hypnosis (p.141) should support your physical and etheric body through this process.

If you have come to the end of this chart without finding any questions that address your particular situation, you may need professional help to achieve an understanding of your addictive problem. Consult your doctor or an association, such as Alcoholics Anonymous, which specializes in addictive behaviours.

Ear acupuncture

In ear acupuncture needles are inserted into the parts of the ear that represent the part of the body that needs treatment. There is also a special "addiction" point. Special studs may be left in this point and massaged to give extra stimulation whenever craving mounts. Electroacupuncture is also used to treat addictions. A small electrical current is passed between needles inserted into each ear, which feels like a gentle buzzing. The endorphin release is thought to provide a natural high, replacing the one that the addictive substance was providing. This can be done as regular sessions or with a portable machine to use, as cravings indicate.

HEADACHES AND MIGRAINES/1

Tension headaches are not the same as migraines, though they may have similar causes. Typically migraines are one-sided, with pain in the eye area and they interfere with daily life. Visual upsets, nausea, and vomiting are also typical. Headaches which last for days, but which do not affect daily life, are usually tension-type headaches.

1 Do you have poor posture, or a past history of back, neck, or lower limb injury, or have you had dental or jaw problems? ▶ **NO** ▶

▼
YES
▼

Headaches and migraines are often associated with misalignment of the spine, pelvis, or skull bones. This is primarily affecting the physical body, but once in place it affects the etheric and sometimes even the emotional bodies.
Class 1 therapies should be helpful, as not only do they treat the physical body but they also affect the etheric and even the emotional body.

2 Do you get headaches or migraines after driving, or after working at a desk, or on a computer? ▶ **NO** ▶

▼
YES
▼

Your posture and vision may be to blame.
Try supportive measures such as regular, simple stretches first, to help relieve tension building at the physical level in your neck and shoulder muscles. Class 1 therapies should be helpful as not only do they treat the physical body but also the etheric and even the emotional body. If these methods do not work, rejoin the chart.

3 Do you get headaches or migraines after missing meals, or replacing meals with sweets or snacks? ▶ **NO** ▶ ▶ ▶

▼
YES
▼

You may be suffering from hypoglycemia or a food sensitivity (see chart, p. 180), indicating a problem in the physical and etheric bodies. You may need to look at physically supportive treatments first. Focus on dietary, food allergy, and supplement treatments.
Once you have addressed these, Class 2 or 8 therapies, which work primarily on the etheric body, may complete your cure. If these methods do not help or are too restrictive, rejoin the chart.

WARNING

See your doctor before following this chart if you are now regularly getting headaches and you previously did not experience them.

Are you drinking enough?

Do you drink at least 1.5 litres (2.5 pints) of water daily? Relative dehydration can be a simple cause of headache and migraine. If you drink caffeine, alcohol, or sugary drinks your need for water will be even higher, as all these other drinks tend to dehydrate. Try drinking 1.5 litres (2.5 pints) water per day together with starting whatever therapy you choose.

4

▶ Do your headaches or migraines seem to be precipitated by head colds or catarrh?

▶ **NO** ▶

▼

YES

▼

The headaches or migraines are probably secondary to this under-lying problem.
See Catarrh and sinus problems chart (p.122).

5

Are you a woman, and do you get headaches or migraines before menstruating, or at other fixed times in your menstrual cycle, or are you approaching the menopause?

▶ **NO** ▶

▼

YES

▼

The headaches or migraines are being triggered by menstrual hormonal changes. This is most obviously happening at the physical and etheric level.
Therapies from Classes 2 and 8 affect the etheric body strongly and Class 3 therapies affect all the subtle bodies. See also PMS chart, p.159.

6

Are you a woman, and have your headaches or migraines started since taking oral contraceptives or hormone replacement therapy (HRT)?

▶ **NO** ▶

go to next page

▼

YES

▼

These cause artificial upsets to the menstrual hormone cycle. Consult your doctor to see if there is a more harmonious preparation. Otherwise it is best not to use these medications, as this side effect is an indication that your physical and etheric bodies are not coping well with the drug.

Work and headaches

Long hours, especially at a computer, trigger headaches in many people. This can be minimized. The main points to check are:

• Vision: If you have not had your eyes tested in the past year, do so.

• Lighting: Light your workspace to avoid glare on the screen. Avoid sitting under a downlight. Make sure that your screen is clean and adjusted to minimize flicker. Position it two feet (60cm) away.

• Seating: Your chair should be the height that you would be to play the piano. Your feet should be on a footrest if necessary, to take the pressure off the backs of the thighs. The small of the back needs support.

• Breaks: For the sake of your back and neck, get up every hour and take a stretch, hunch your shoulders, and then relax. Spend a couple of minutes looking out of the window into the distance, or cup your eyes in your hands.

• Drinks: Take plenty of water. Air-conditioning and computers are dehydrating, making you more prone to headaches.

• Phones: If you have to use the phone and computer simultaneously, hold the phone in your hand, not in your neck, or use a neck rest.

HEADACHES AND MIGRAINES/2

7

a) Do you develop your headaches or migraines at the weekend?

▶ NO ▶

▼
YES
▼

b) Do you drink more tea/coffee on weekdays (at work), than at home at weekends?

▶ NO ▶

▼
YES
▼

Your symptoms may be due to caffeine withdrawal.
Cut out tea, coffee, cola, and chocolate for 1 month. Caffeine affects the etheric as well as the physical body, as it fools us into feeling we have more energy at our disposal than we really have.

8

Do you develop headaches or migraines when confronted with a deadline or a period of intense activity?

▼
YES
▼

The stress of your task is channeling itself into neck and shoulder tension. Your work posture may be aggravating this physically. The stress is triggering belief systems in the mental body, going on to activate an emotional response which you are repressing by holding it as tension in the physical body. It is important to learn how to relax. *Try a therapy from Class 11, or better, try a Class 4 therapy, helping you to use your body in a more relaxed way. Class 5 and 6 therapies will help you express emotional responses more clearly and release you from belief inhibitions. If none of these methods is of use or appeals to you, rejoin the chart.*

9

▶ NO ▶ Do you find it difficult to unwind or relax?

▼
YES
▼

This is probably a habit pattern you have developed in the mental body. It immediately affects the emotional, etheric, and physical bodies.
A relaxation technique method such as from Class 4, 11, or 12 should be useful.

▶ NO ▶ ▶ ▶

► ► Do you find it difficult to express your emotions either verbally or physically?

▼

YES

▼

This is likely to be upsetting your emotional body and leading to physical tension.
Techniques to help your emotional body express itself more clearly can be used from Classes 5, 6, and 11.

► NO ►  Do you get headaches or migraines after, or instead of, arguments?

▼

YES

▼

The headache is probably because your emotional body is unable to express itself freely. This may be due to your external circumstances, but it is more likely to be due to your own beliefs about how you or others should behave – a mental body problem.
Try Class 5, 6, and 7 therapies to give you the opportunity to allow your physical and emotional bodies to express themselves more freely. Class 11 therapies will help you work with your emotional and mental bodies.

► NO ► Is there altogether too much going on in your life – good or bad?

▼

YES

▼

Your causal body is probably trying to get you to make some quiet space in your life. This may be impossible and you may need to resort temporarily to supportive drug treatments. However symptoms indicate that your stress is too much for you, so therapies to help you handle it are beneficial. All your subtle bodies are being affected.
*Massage from Class 1, shiatsu from Class 2, or techniques from Classes 3, 4, 5 , 6 , 7, 10, and 11 are all good, depending on personal preferences.
All give an opportunity to move into a quieter, deeper space, which helps bring balance into your life and may reduce the "need" for migraines to "quiet" you.
Also meditation (Class 12) is recommended for its ability to relax you and connect you more consciously to your causal body.*

► NO ►

go to next page

HEADACHES AND MIGRAINES/3

⑬

Are you a "born worrier"? ▸NO▸

▼

YES

▼

Worrying is the result of problems in the mental body, resulting from a faulty belief system. The effects filter into the emotional, etheric, and physical bodies so that none can function freely.

It is important to learn how to relax, so try a Class 4 or 11 therapy. However, to change the need for worry is more fundamental. Also consider Class 3, 8, and 12 therapies, which may help you to change your belief system.

⑭

Have you recently moved house or job location, though neither causes obvious stress? ▸NO▸

▼

YES

▼

Your home, especially your bedroom or your workplace, may be carrying environmental stress of some type. Asking others in the same environment if they have health problems might clarify the situation.

Look at Class 9 and 10 techniques as these focus on healing the environment or altering the effect the environment has on your subtle bodies.

⑮

a) Do you develop headaches the day after drinking alcohol? ▸NO▸ ▸ ▸

▼

YES

▼

b) Have you drunk more than 3 units of alcohol when this happens? ▸NO▸

▼

YES

▼

c) Would you answer "yes" to 2 or more of these questions: ▸NO▸ ▸ ▸
● Do you ever worry about how much you are drinking?
● Have others ever expressed concern about the amount you drink?
● Have you been late for work or missed work because of hangover headaches?
● Do you ever feel guilty about the amount you drink?

▼

YES

▼

Your alcohol intake may be a source of addiction for you.
See Addiction chart (p.141).

ORTHODOX TREATMENTS – HEADACHES

A simple headache usually improves after taking a painkiller such as aspirin, paracetamol, or a non-steroidal anti-inflammatory drug (NSAID). This is available in a low-dose over-the-counter painkiller. Preparations containing codeine or caffeine are prescribed for headaches and some of these are available over the counter. These can have a stronger effect, but if you are a regular sufferer avoid them because when you stop taking them you are likely to suffer a rebound or a withdrawal headache, compounding the original problem. Also these drugs are addictive. If you suffer from frequent headaches your doctor may diagnose them as tension headaches. Recent research indicates that they are due to tension building up in the neck and shoulders, which sets up muscle spasm at the base of the skull. This affects the thin sheet of muscle that covers the whole of the scalp. It is this pulling on the scalp that causes the pain.

Tension headaches are surprisingly hard to treat; the best treatment in orthodox medicine is a NSAID-type painkiller. These drugs often cause digestive side effects, sometimes serious, such as bleeding from the stomach. Because of the difficulty of treating this apparently simple problem many people turn to complementary medicine, with good results in many cases.

▶ ▶ ▶ ▶ ▶ ▶ ▶ ▶ ▶ ▶ ▶ ▶

16

Do headaches or migraines run in your family?

▼

YES

▼

You may have inherited a weakness that makes you prone to headaches. This may be at the mental or emotional level, but most likely at the etheric level. *Choose a method that works on all these levels, but especially the etheric, such as Class 2, 8, and 14 therapies.*

▶ ▶ Either the amount you are drinking or the type of alcohol you are drinking does not suit you. Try cutting down or changing to another type of alcohol. Drink plenty of water before bed. Avoid a hangover by taking 5 evening primrose capsules, 2 high-dose vitamin B complex, and eating something starchy or fatty before drinking. However the hangover is a sign that your physical body is not happy with alcohol and it would be best to avoid it.

17

▶ NO ▶ Have you tried a manipulation therapy for your headaches, as well as other approaches to treatment?

▼

YES

▼

If you have reached the end of this chart without identifying a cause, the original cause may have gone, but the etheric body is still responding in an illness pattern. Try a Class 2, 8, or 14 therapy. These primarily work on the etheric body, which may be holding the symptoms in place. If none of these helps, look inside yourself to find out what the headache or migraine might represent. Deep changes in consciousness may be trying to take place. Therapies most likely to be beneficial are those that help connect you to your causal body. Classes 3, 7, 11, and 12 are particularly good for this.

◀ ◀ ◀ ◀ ◀ ◀ ◀ ◀ ◀ ◀

▼

Your attempts to cure your headaches may be hampered by the continuation of long-standing disturbances of the spine, especially in the upper spine and pelvis, that continue to undermine the other work you are doing. *Try a Class 1 therapy to realign both your physical and etheric body.*

▶ NO ▾

see below

▾ ▾

ORTHODOX TREATMENTS – MIGRAINES

Migraines are notoriously difficult to treat with orthodox drugs and the most effective treatments are prone to unpleasant side effects. If simple headache remedies do not work the next group of drugs used are painkillers combined with an anti-nausea drug or an anti-histamine. The treatment needs to be started at the first indication, though some migraines do not respond. There are now other drugs that may help. One group is ergotamines, which can cause serious side effects, especially if taken too often. There is also a new group of drugs that affect serotonin levels. These are very effective in true migraine, but cause odd side effects such as enhancing pain elsewhere, sore throat, tingling, and excess urination. For sufferers of frequent migraines there is a number of drugs that can be taken daily to prevent them, for example small doses of either beta-blockers or antidepressants. Migraines are so incapacitating and the drug treatments so prone to side effects that sufferers are strongly motivated to try complementary treatments.

BACK AND NECK PAIN/1

①

a) Is your back/neck pain either long-standing or recurrent?

▶ **NO** ▶ You may have triggered reflex muscle spasm in the spinal muscles by injuring your back, overuse, or by using it awkwardly, or by sleeping awkwardly. *See also ★ below, right.*

▼
YES
▼

b) Have you suffered from whiplash or other back injuries in the past?

▶ **NO** ▶

②

Has your back pain been present since giving birth?

▶ **NO** ▶

③

Has your back pain existed since having an operation?

▶ **NO** ▶ ▶ ▶

▼
YES
▼

See ★ right.

▼
YES
▼

See ★ right.

▼
YES
▼

★ Usually this problem is due to slight misalignments of one or more of the small "facet" joints that protrude from each vertebra. It is less common for the disc linking the vertebrae to be the cause – this produces more symptoms (see warning, below). Relaxation of the spinal muscles is often enough to allow the facets to slip back into alignment. This can also be achieved by adjusting the facets directly. The problem is at the etheric and physical level. *Treatments that directly affect these levels are Class 1 and 2 therapies.*

ORTHODOX TREATMENTS

Back pain is one of the commonest causes of debility and is poorly handled by orthodox medicine. Most acute back problems clear up on their own over a two- to six-week period. During that time painkillers, which may have unpleasant or serious side effects in themselves, are the usual treatment. Chronic or recurrent back problems can be very difficult to treat successfully. Basic back care and painkillers are still the main treatments.

Back surgery and chronic pain management are the last resorts in treatment.

Conventional medicine has shown that other methods, in particular chiropractic, are better at helping back pain than orthodox methods, but such treatments are not readily available. For these reasons many people turn to complementary therapists for help.

WARNING

If you are experiencing weakness or numbness in any limb, or problems with passing faeces or urine, see your doctor. Your pain may have a more serious underlying cause such as a slipped disc or, very rarely, a growth pressing on the spinal cord.

Chronic pain

If you have had endless treatments for back pain and are now wondering whether you are ever going to be free of it, whatever your problem was initially, you are now probably suffering from pain coming directly from irritated nerves.

4

▶ NO ▶ Are you over 40 years of age and have you had spinal X rays done that "explain" why you have back pain?

▼

YES

▼

Check with your doctor what these results really mean. Indications of osteoarthritis, loss of joint space, and signs of degeneration are as common in back pain sufferers as non-sufferers. Even with such X rays you can still be completely pain-free. The pain is due to nerve and muscle contraction rather than bone problems. Treatments at the etheric and physical level may help.
Consider Class 1, 2, and 6 treatments. Class 4 methods also work at these levels and provide a discipline to keep your back strong and flexible, making you less prone to a recurrence of pain.

5

▶ NO ▶ How is your posture? Do you have an exceptionally long back, or exaggerated curves at the waist or neck? Are you unusually straight at the waist or neck? Are your shoulders uneven?

▼

YES

▼

All these are distortions from the natural curves and symmetry of the spine. Also, after time, back problems create their own distortions, producing a vicious circle of distortion and pain. Improving your posture can make a real difference. Posture is not just a disturbance at the physical and etheric levels, often the emotional body is involved.
Class 1 and 2 therapies help relieve pain and improve posture, but if there is a large emotional component – repressed emotions or unhelpful attitudes – Class 6 and even Class 11 psycho-therapeutic methods are useful. To help maintain and strengthen posture consider Class 4 techniques.

6

▶ NO ▶ Are you weight-training? ▶ NO ▶

▼

YES

▼

Unequal development of muscle bulk can distress the spine and trap spinal nerves, causing pain. *Class 1, 2, and 6 therapies can relieve this pain at the physical and etheric level. A Class 4 discipline, which develops balance and flexibility alongside your weight-training, will help prevent this problem from recurring.*

go to next page

BACK AND NECK PAIN/2

7

Do you feel that:
● You are weighed down by responsibilities?
● You are unsupported in what you do?
● You are putting up with a lot from life or from other people?

▼

YES

▼

These feelings are all responses to stress and relate particularly to the spine's role in the emotional as well as the physical body. Your back pain may be the "acting out" of your feelings. The emotional body is affecting the etheric and physical body and treatments that act at all these levels are useful.
Consider Class 6 therapies. These are able to access the emotional body and help release trapped energy levels. Class 11 psycho-therapy is also useful, in conjunction with Class 1 and 2 therapies. Together they help release energy from the etheric body by bringing repressed emotions to the surface, helping you to relax and change your attitudes, so that you can handle stress in a healthier way. Class 3 and 12 methods are also helpful because they align all your subtle bodies with your causal body.

▸ NO ▸

8

Do you suffer from a number of niggling symptoms as well as back pain – none of which your doctor can really help?

▼

YES

▼

You may be suffering from food allergies.
See Food sensitivities chart (p.180).

▸ NO ▸

9

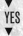

Do you have sleep problems, or low energy, as though life is tedious or hard work?

▼

YES

▼

Chronic back pain can cause these symptoms of depression, but sometimes depression is the primary problem. Whatever came first, resolving the depression can be the way to help relieve the back pain.
See Depression chart (p.136).

◂ ◂ ◂ ◂ ◂ ◂ ◂ ◂ ◂ ◂

▼

If you have come to the end of this chart without finding an approach to help you deal with your back pain, see your doctor again. It may be that your back pain is secondary to another condition such as a gynaecological or digestive problem and this may need further investigation.

▸ NO ▼

see below

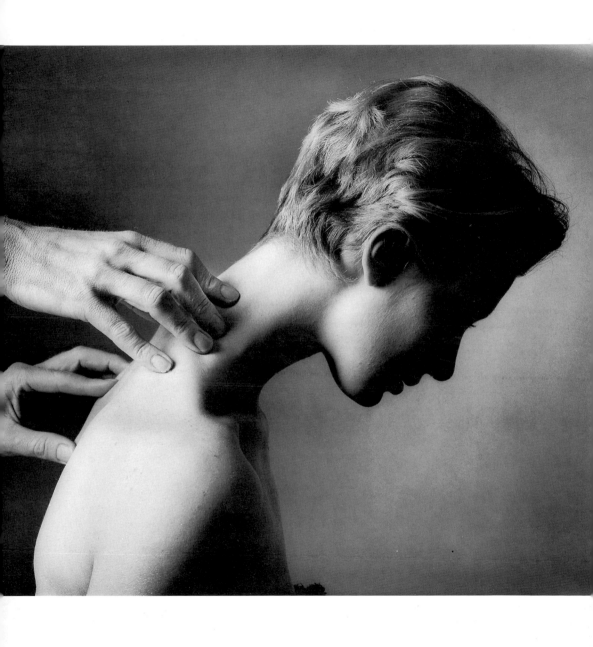

ARTHRITIS AND RHEUMATISM/1

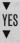 **1**

Are you a woman suffering from menopausal symptoms?

▼ **YES**
▼

Non-specific aches and pains can be a menopausal symptom. *See Menopause chart (p.167).*

▸ **NO** ▸ **2**

Do you have a number of unrelated symptoms as well as your arthritis/rheumatism?

▼ **YES**
▼

If you have not seen your doctor, do so before continuing this chart. If your doctor is not able to come up with a diagnosis you may be suffering from food sensitivities. *See Food sensitivities chart (p.180).*

▸ **NO** ▸ **3**

Do you have various aches and pains that you put down to getting older?

▼ **YES**
▼

This is very common and often accompanied by loss of flexibility and strength. As we age exercise becomes increasingly important, to maintain strength and flexibility. *Disciplines that help achieve and maintain this are Class 4 techniques. These work both at the physical and etheric level. They also help by retraining you to use your body more efficiently. Class 6 techniques are also helpful. Increasing strength, flexibility, and efficiency of the body can help relieve arthritis symptoms. Sometimes dietary changes, herbs, or food supplements can help aches and pains. Consider also a Class 14 approach. This helps at the etheric and physical level.*

▸ **NO** ▸ ▸ ▸

4

▶ ▶ Have you suffered an injury to your arthritic joint(s) in the past?

▶ NO ▶ Does rheumatism/ arthritis run in your family?

▶ NO ▶ Do you have difficulties expressing emotion, particularly anger, or do you experience resentment at being overworked?

▶ NO ▶

go to next page

▼

YES

▼

Injury to a joint makes it prone to injury in later life. Some of this is due to the function of not only the joint but the rest of the musculoskeletal system being disturbed.

Therapies that help re-align the system, such as Class 1, 2, or 6 treatments, can help restore muscular balance in the body. This can relieve the stress on an arthritic joint. These treatments work mainly at the etheric and physical level.

▼

YES

▼

You have probably inherited a tendency to arthritis. Energy healing can affect these tendencies by working with the etheric body, in particular. This carries the genetic blueprint.

Physically supportive therapies that include diet, herbs, and/or supplements are also useful. Consider Class 2, 8, and 14 therapies, which are able to help the etheric body.

▼

YES

▼

The physical body can "act out" inner feelings.

If you feel this may be a problem consider a Class 6 therapy which uses the body to access and release these feelings. If expression is difficult, consider a Class 5 therapy to help you move into expressing these feelings creatively. Class 7 therapies also release trapped emotion.

If you like to work with your mind, Class 11 psychotherapies can be useful. If resentment and forgiveness are problems consider a Class 3 therapy.

ARTHRITIS AND RHEUMATISM/2

7

Has your arthritis been given a specific diagnosis, such as rheumatoid arthritis or gout?

▶ **NO** ▶ *If you cannot find helpful guidelines from this chart see your doctor to check that arthritis/rheumatism is the problem. Once you have done that, consider Class 2, 8, or 14 therapies, which generally help this condition by acting on the etheric body. If these do not help, your symptoms may be an indication that you need to look more deeply at your life. A major shift in consciousness may be called for. Class 3, 11, or 12 therapies, which can connect you more deeply with your causal self, may be useful to achieve this.*

▼

YES

▼

These types of arthritis are diseases in themselves and may need orthodox medication to limit joint damage. However energy healing can be very beneficial. *Consider Class 2, 8, and 14 therapies, which have a strong effect on the etheric body, where the disease first manifests.*

ORTHODOX TREATMENTS

For some forms of arthritis, such as rheumatoid arthritis and gout, there is a range of medical treatments that can improve a person's quality of life, though they do not actually cure the disease. The treatment of the commonest form of arthritis, osteoarthritis, is almost entirely pain relief. The mainstay for the treatment of arthritis is the use of painkilling drugs, in particular non-steroidal anti-inflammatory drugs (NSAIDs) such as ibuprofen. Other treatments include steroids that are injected into the most painful area of the joint.

Unfortunately all drugs can produce side effects, some of which can be serious, and some painkillers, such as codeine-based preparations, can also be addictive. Surgery, such as hip replacement, can help by replacing very damaged joints, but such operations require intense rehabilitation. This can be daunting for elderly patients. For these reasons many people turn to energy-healing methods for help.

PRE-MENSTRUAL SYNDROME/1

The term "pre-menstrual syndrome", or PMS, covers up to 150 different symptoms, which occur regularly at the same time in the cycle and are relieved once menstruation is over. It is thought that imbalances in progesterone and oestrogen are to blame.

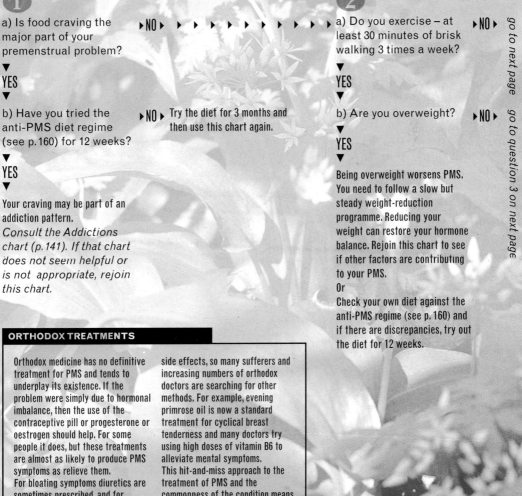

1

a) Is food craving the major part of your premenstrual problem? ▶NO ▶ ▶ ▶ ▶ ▶ ▶ ▶ ▶ ▶ ▶ ▶

▼
YES
▼

b) Have you tried the anti-PMS diet regime (see p. 160) for 12 weeks? ▶NO ▶ Try the diet for 3 months and then use this chart again.

▼
YES
▼

Your craving may be part of an addiction pattern.
Consult the Addictions chart (p. 141). If that chart does not seem helpful or is not appropriate, rejoin this chart.

2

a) Do you exercise – at least 30 minutes of brisk walking 3 times a week? ▶NO ▶

▼
YES
▼

b) Are you overweight? ▶NO ▶

▼
YES
▼

Being overweight worsens PMS. You need to follow a slow but steady weight-reduction programme. Reducing your weight can restore your hormone balance. Rejoin this chart to see if other factors are contributing to your PMS.
Or
Check your own diet against the anti-PMS regime (see p. 160) and if there are discrepancies, try out the diet for 12 weeks.

go to next page

go to question 3 on next page

ORTHODOX TREATMENTS

Orthodox medicine has no definitive treatment for PMS and tends to underplay its existence. If the problem were simply due to hormonal imbalance, then the use of the contraceptive pill or progesterone or oestrogen should help. For some people it does, but these treatments are almost as likely to produce PMS symptoms as relieve them.
For bloating symptoms diuretics are sometimes prescribed, and for anxiety or depression symptoms anti-depressants and tranquillizers are sometimes used. Using drugs in this way to treat PMS is a very superficial approach and not without side effects, so many sufferers and increasing numbers of orthodox doctors are searching for other methods. For example, evening primrose oil is now a standard treatment for cyclical breast tenderness and many doctors try using high doses of vitamin B6 to alleviate mental symptoms.
This hit-and-miss approach to the treatment of PMS and the commonness of the condition means that huge numbers of women have tried alternative treatments of some sort. The dietary and nutritional supplement approach is popular and can be successful.

PRE-MENSTRUAL SYNDROME/2

▸ ▸

▸ ▸ ▸ a) Do your symptoms make you feel that your lifestyle or family situation is intolerable?

▸NO▸

▼

YES

▼

b) Do you, to a lesser extent, still feel this way once the PMS is over?

▸NO▸

▼

YES

▼

go to question 4 (next page)

PMS is an indication from your subconscious that all is not well. *A psychotherapeutic approach, such as a Class 11 therapy, can help you fully reveal what is not working in your present way of being and help you express feelings more freely. These therapies access the mental and emotional bodies and released energy filters through to the etheric and physical bodies. Also these therapies can help connect you with your causal body. Class 3 therapies help align your subtle bodies. Class 4 and 12 meditation techniques also help to achieve this alignment and reconnect you to your causal body.*

▸ Lack of exercise can worsen PMS. For the next 3 months increase your exercise to at least 30 minutes' brisk walk 3 times a week. Some therapies combine physical exercise with work on the subtle bodies. These would be particularly helpful. *Class 4 therapies provide exercise at the physical level, but free up and align all the subtle bodies at the same time. Class 5 therapies provide much freer exercise and also greatly enhance connection to the emotional body. This helps release problems held at the emotional level, which filter down to the physical and etheric bodies. If these therapies do not appeal or do not work, rejoin this chart.*

12-week anti-PMS regime

Try this for three cycles, or use it in combination with an energy-based treatment. Diet changes work on the physical body to affect primarily the physical body, but these changes permeate to the subtle bodies. Mental clarity and emotional stability can both be affected by dietary changes and psychics can see changes in the aura brought about simply by changes in diet. So at some level, apparently physical "treatments" affect the subtle bodies.

- Limit consumption of caffeine, salt, sugar, red meat, fats, alcohol, and dairy foods.
- If you smoke – stop.
- Increase intake of fibre, aiming for 5 portions of vegetables, salad, or fruits daily.
- Eat regular meals.
- Don't skimp on protein. It is not needed in large amounts, but many women eat too little.

4

a) Do you feel that you have enough time for yourself?

▼
YES
▼

▶NO▶ b) Do you feel that you are not receiving enough touch or care?

▼
YES
▼

Touch and being cared for is essential for wellbeing. Our physical, etheric, and emotional bodies become energetically disturbed without it.
Class 1 massage-type therapies and Class 2 shiatsu, reflexology, and Class 6 therapies help by relieving tension in the etheric body and trapped emotion in the emotional body. Class 3 hands-on healing techniques can also help by realigning all the subtle bodies.

▶NO▶ c) Have you lost your creative urges or ability to "play"?

▼
YES
▼

Creativity and play naturally restore energy balance in the subtle bodies. Give yourself time to encourage and renew your creativity.
Class 5 therapies can be very useful. They use the physical body to increase and balance the energy flow, particularly in the emotional and etheric bodies.

▶NO▼

go to question 5 (below)

5

Did your PMS symptoms replace painful and/or heavy menstruation, or did your PMS follow childbirth? Or have you had PMS ever since your menarche?

▼
YES
▼

See ★ right.

▶NO▶ Are your PMS symptoms mainly physical, such as tender breasts?

▼
YES
▼

★ Changes in your hormonal balance may have triggered the PMS. Hormones affect the etheric and physical bodies.
Treatments that work at these levels are helpful, for example Class 2, 8, and 14 therapies.

▶NO▶ Are you approaching the menopause?

▼
YES
▼

PMS symptoms can merge into perimenopausal symptoms – see the Menopause chart (p. 167).

▶NO▶

go to question 8a (next page)

PRE-MENSTRUAL SYNDROME/3

8

a) Do you find it easy to get in touch with your feelings?

▶NO ▶ ▶ ▶ ▶ ▶ ▶ ▶ ▶ ▶ ▶ ▶ ▶

▼ YES ▼

b) Did your **PMS** occur in the months following moving to a new home, a new bedroom? Or redecorating a main room in your home, especially your bedroom?

▶NO ▶

▼ YES ▼

These changes may have disrupted your relationship to your environment at a subtle level. Environments and colours both influence the body energy fields. *If a move to a new home has triggered a problem, consider Class 9 or 13 treatments. These can also help neutralize the effects the environment is having on your etheric and emotional bodies, which are most affected by these energies. Class 10 colour therapy may also be useful to help choose more appropriate colour schemes.*

If you cannot find a cause for your PMS symptoms from this chart, recheck with your doctor that your symptoms are due to PMS. Otherwise try a Class 2, 8, or 14 therapy, which work on the etheric body. Hormones have an effect here and can be rebalanced at this level. If this does not help then look inside yourself more deeply to find out what PMS may represent, with reference to your belief systems and mental body. The problem may be that you are having difficulties making changes in your beliefs that are preventing deep changes in consciousness from happening. Such changes have the potential to affect all your subtle bodies as well as the physical body. The therapies most likely to help in this process are ones that connect you to your causal body. Class 3, 7, 11, and 12 therapies are all particularly helpful in this process.

▶ The PMS may be the end result of trapped energy in the emotional body. Treatments that will help clear this and free up emotions should help.
Class 5, 6, and 7 methods, which work on the physical body to access the emotional body, can be useful and do not need you to think about your emotional state. Class 11 is also useful, as these therapies approach the problem from the psychological angle.

PROBLEM MENSTRUATION/1

1

Has your doctor told you
that there is a structural
explanation for your
symptoms?

▸NO▸

▼

YES

▼

*See General advice box
(p.164), and follow your
doctor's advice.*

2

Is your problem
menstruation associated
with symptoms of
premenstrual tension?

▸NO▸

▼

YES

▼

See PMS chart, p.159.

3

Has your menstruation
been painful and/or heavy
ever since your menarche?

▸NO▸

▼

YES

▼

This is due to the cycle of
hormones triggered at the
menarche having not settled
down into a balanced pattern.
A method that affects the etheric
body can be useful.
*Consider a Class 2, 8, or 14
therapy.*

go to next page

ORTHODOX TREATMENTS

If a specific cause is found, such as
fibroids or endometriosis, orthodox
medicine uses either drugs or
surgery for treatment.
At one time hysterectomy was used
extensively to eliminate menstrual
problems. This is successful in
removing the problem, but it also
removes childbearing ability and,
for some women, a sense of femi-
ninity. Such radical treatment for
benign conditions is used less and
less and drugs are being used more.
Sex hormones, in the form of the
contraceptive pill, and progesterone
as tablets or in the progesterone
coil, are particularly useful. The
anti-inflammatory drug mefenamic
acid is used both for painful and
heavy bleeding and new drugs that
affect clotting may also help.
However, there may be problems
with side effects and the
treatments themselves are not
curative in most situations. The
use of the contraceptive pill for
adolescent menstrual pains and
endometriosis can be exceptions.

PROBLEM MENSTRUATION/2

4

Do you know or suspect that you might have suffered some sexual trauma earlier in your life?

▸NO▸

▼
YES
▼

This is a very difficult area and needs highly skilled attention. Your emotional body may have been affected and this can filter through to the etheric and physical bodies.
Class 11 psychotherapeutic techniques are a good approach. This can combine well with Class 3 light-touch techniques, which can help balance all the subtle bodies.

5

Does painful and/or heavy menstruation run in your family?

▸NO▸

▼
YES
▼

This may be an inherited tendency, likely to be found in the etheric body.
Therapies that primarily act at the etheric level, such as Class 2 and 8 therapies, may be useful. Class 14 therapies are also helpful.

6

Are you approaching the menopause?

▸NO▸ ▸ ▸ ▸

▼
YES
▼

The disturbance in hormone balance that precedes the menopause often disrupts the menstrual cycle.
For self-help and advice at this time see the Menopause chart (p.167).

General advice

Painful or heavy menstruation from adolescence is usually hormonal in cause. But as women age there is more likely to be a physical cause that can be detected by physical examination. It is most important that you see your doctor before using this chart. However, if a physical cause is found, you can still use the chart, as many of the physical causes of bleeding or pain have an underlying hormonal cause, which can be influenced by energy-based therapies.
Your doctor can check for anaemia, which causes heavier menstruation. But don't start iron supplements without blood tests, as taking iron when you don't need to can disturb the absorption of other minerals.

7

▸ ▸ Has your menstruation been heavier and/or more painful since childbirth?

▾

YES

▾

Go to question 8.

▸NO▸ **8**

Was the birth traumatic or else have you been left with backache, headaches, or pains down your legs?

▾

YES

▾

The trauma of the birth may have disrupted the alignment of the pelvis. This might be something physical preventing the free flow of energy in the etheric body that goes with healthy hormonal functioning.

A Class 1 therapy that works on the physical but also affects the etheric body might be useful. This can combine well with Class 3 light-touch therapies, and Class 2 therapies, which help at the etheric body level directly.

▸NO▸ **9**

Do you feel you have had enough time and attention for yourself since the birth of your child?

▾

YES

▾

Pregnancy, childbirth, and breast-feeding all require complex changes in the subtle balance of hormones. This affects the etheric as well as the physical body. You may not have adjusted as well as you might to all these changes. *Try a Class 2, 8, or 14 therapy, which works on the etheric body, to help readjust your hormones.*

Go to question 10 (next page).

◂ ◂ ◂ ◂ ◂ ◂ ◂ ◂ ◂ ◂

▾

Although there is likely to be a hormonal upset that is disturbing the physical level, the problem is in the emotional body. This part of the subtle body responds greatly to touch and your etheric body also responds to this.

Try an enjoyable touch-orientated therapy such as massage or aromatherapy from Class 1, or a Class 6 therapy. Class 3 light-touch techniques, although more subtle, can also be helpful.

Go to question 10 (next page).

▸NO▾

see below

10

Did your menstruation problems follow an injury to your back, neck, or head?

▼

YES

▼

There may be a structural problem in your pelvis that is disturbing the energy flow at the level of the etheric body. Your injury could have caused this. *Try a Class 1 therapy, which works directly on the physical level but also influences the etheric body.*

▸NO▸

11

Do you get back or leg pains with your difficult menstruation?

▼

YES

▼

There may be an energy blockage at the etheric level in your pelvis. Underlying this may be a structural problem that may require orthodox treatment. *However therapies that deal with both the etheric and the physical level may be helpful. Consider a Class 1, 2, or 6 therapy.*

▸NO▸

12

Have your menstruation problems arisen since moving house or changing to a different bedroom?

▼

YES

▼

Hormones are very sensitive to subtle changes in the environment. It is possible that you have picked up some disturbance in your environment. *To correct this consider a Class 9, 10, or 13 technique. These are able to influence the subtle energies of your environment and protect you against their effects.*

▸NO▾

see below

◂ ◂ ◂ ◂ ◂ ◂ ◂ ◂ ◂ ▾

If you cannot find a cause, consult your doctor to check there is no physical cause. Otherwise try a Class 2, 8, or 14 therapy, which work with the etheric body. Hormones have an effect here and can be rebalanced at this level. If this does not help you may need to look more deeply within to find out what your problems represent with reference to your belief systems and mental body. You may be having difficulties making a change in your beliefs to allow a deep change in consciousness. Such changes can affect all your subtle bodies as well as the physical. Consider therapies that help you consciously connect to your causal body. Class 3, 7, 8, 11, and 12 therapies are all particularly helpful.

MENOPAUSE/1

The menopause is not an illness, though in Western society it has been considered so for centuries. Over 89 per cent of women experience significant symptoms (see box, p.169). On average menopause occurs at about 52 years of age, though it can happen in the thirties and, very occasionally, earlier. Not all menopausal changes are due to hormones – for example, weight gain and ageing.

Are the physical discomforts of the menopause your chief worry?

▸ **NO** ▸

▼
YES
▼
▼

▸ ▸ ▸ ▸ ▸ ▸ ▸ ▸ ▸ ▸

Are you happy with your lifestyle and enjoy life, but find mood changes and/or memory and concentration a problem?

▸ **NO** ▸

▼
YES
▼

These symptoms are direct effects on your physical body of the fluctuating oestrogen levels that precede the menopause. These symptoms start as the menopause approaches and fade afterwards. Two years is an average time for this to settle. You may want to consider HRT. If you cannot tolerate HRT or are looking for a more natural approach, herbalism and nutritional supplements can help at the physical and etheric levels (see Diet and the menopause box, p.169).

On a directly energetic level, treatments that act on the etheric body are useful. Consider a Class 2 or 8 therapy. Class 14 also looks at physical support measures. There is no reason why you should not combine several of these approaches.

Do heart disease, strokes, or osteoporosis run in your family? Or do you suffer from diabetes or a chronic disease such as rheumatoid arthritis, for which you have had prolonged treatment with steroids?

▸ **NO** ▸

▼
YES
▼

Current understanding of HRT indicates that its use maintains natural protection against heart disease and possibly osteoporosis. Unfortunately this only continues while HRT is being used. If you are in this "at risk" category, consider making lifestyle and dietary changes to help protect against these diseases. Your doctor can provide information. As energy-healing methods can work to both prevent and treat illnesses they can be very useful.

Class 2 and 8 therapies work on the etheric body and can affect the physical body through this. Class 4 therapies, particularly yoga and tai chi, are also excellent to help maintain fitness and health into old age. These act at all levels of the subtle body. A supplement and/or nutritional approach is also useful, e.g. a Class 14 therapy.

go to next page

MENOPAUSE/2

④

Are you feeling a loss or self-esteem – losing your looks or sexuality, or feeling you have spent your whole life as a mother and are fit for nothing else?

▸ NO ▸

▾
YES
▾

External changes are having a much greater effect on you than is actually the case. It is unlikely that others are noticing these changes. You are responding to the menopause as a loss, whereas it is a move to a different phase of life.
See also ★ right

⑤

Do you feel, or would you like to feel, that the menopause signifies the end of an old way of life and the start of a new phase?

▸ NO ▸ ▸ ▸ ▸ ▸ ▸ ▸ ▸ ▸ ▸ ▸ ▸ ▸ ▸ ▸ ▸

▾
YES
▾

★ After the menopause there is a change in the nature of a woman's creativity. Women become free to be creative in their own right and can use the wisdom gained in the childbearing years. For women without children this creativity is often already in place, but the menopause brings it into its own. This can be experienced as a deep sense of "aliveness".
Try a class that most appeals to your sense of joy and exploration. Class 1 massage-type treatments re-establish a connection between your physical and subtle bodies. Class 2

shiatsu and reflexology are also good. Class 3 therapies help similarly, but more subtly, with less emphasis on the physical. If you enjoy discipline Class 4 methods are excellent, but for many the freedom of expression of a Class 5 method opens up the emotional body in a new way. Class 7 methods have a similar effect. A Class 10 therapy, particularly colour therapy, is a good approach for difficulties with appearance. If you like to work with the psychological areas Class 11 therapies in general are helpful. Shamanic-type work is particularly powerful during the menopause. Class 12 meditation is another way of keeping open the connection with the causal body and one's sense of being alive.

ORTHODOX TREATMENTS

Recently there has been an upsurge in hormonal supplement treatment (HRT). For many this removes distressing symptoms. Medical research indicates that the symptoms are due to the irregularity and subsequent fall in oestrogen. Oestrogen seems to protect from heart disease, strokes, and osteoporosis. The downside is that it seems to trigger some cancers. Another problem is that HRT effects only last while the treatment is taken. There is a big debate as to what are the real benefits and risks, what are valid alternatives, and whether this non-disease needs treating anyway. Also, for some, HRT triggers worse side effects than menopausal symptoms.

6

▸ ▸ Are you feeling distanced from your partner and/or family, or do you feel loss of ambition or enthusiasm for your work or former interests?

▾

YES

▾

This is more of a mid-life crisis than a menopausal symptom. Your partner may well be feeling the same. It doesn't mean that you need a new relationship, new job, or new activities, though it might. What is more important is to discover a new way of relating to these aspects of your life. It might also be possible that you have lost touch with who you really are. This deep sense of Self is tied into your energy of being alive and if it becomes blocked tiredness and depression will follow.

Consider techniques that help your causal body – these will increase the flow of energy through all your other subtle bodies as well (e.g. Classes 2, 3, 4, 5, 8, 11, and 12). One common need at this time is for one's own space. This requires re-adjustment rather than a radical shakeup. The re-alignment of your subtle bodies can help you see what you need to do more clearly.

7

▸ NO ▸ Are you consulting this chart because you believe that the menopause, if not an illness, is at least a problem?

▾

YES

▾

You may have naturally adjusted to this change and need not go deeper, but there is no reason why your body has to suffer. It is good to review eating and exercise habits, as getting older implies an increased likelihood of degenerative diseases.
A Class 4 technique is particularly useful to maintain good health into old age, as is meditation (Class 12).

▸ NO ▸ Your symptoms may not be connected with the menopause. Consult your doctor: there may be another cause for your concern.

Symptoms of menopause

• Perimenopausal: Hot flushes, night sweats, disturbed sleep and headaches, mood swings, anxiety, irritability, weak memory and poor concentration, aches and pains.

• Post-menopausal: Thinning of vaginal skin, loss of libido, general thinning of skin and softening of breasts.
• "Invisible" post-menopausal: Susceptibility to heart disease, osteoporosis.

Diet and the menopause

As perimenopausal symptoms are equivalent to an extended period of PMS, the anti-PMS regime (see p. 160) is useful. For many women hot flushes are triggered by caffeine, alcohol, smoking, and spicy foods. After the menopause, bone tends to lose calcium and magnesium, which is the cause of osteoporosis, so these nutrients become especially important in the diet. Dairy foods are rich in calcium, but can cause other problems such as raised cholesterol and weight gain. Calcium-enriched soya products are an alternative. The calcium enables bone metabolism to work maximally and so helps prevent osteoporosis, and the soya mimics oestrogen. Both help the symptoms of the menopause and protect against breast cancer.

EATING DISORDERS/1

①

Do you suffer from anorexia or bulimia?

▶ NO ▶

▼

YES

▼

Therapies that help anorexia and bulimia affect both the mental and emotional bodies, and the etheric and physical body. The illness seems to be a false belief system, often related to physical appearance.
Class 11 therapies, working at the emotional and mental levels, can be useful. Therapies such as Class 2, 8, or 14, which work with the subtle bodies, can be helpful. If you find it difficult to contact or express your feelings verbally, Class 5 techniques can be useful.

②

Do you find yourself vomiting, or taking laxatives or diuretics to keep your weight down?

▶ NO ▶

▼

YES

▼

This is a serious symptom of anorexia/bulimia. See your doctor. You may wish to combine orthodox treatment with complementary therapies. Rejoin the chart for further advice.

③

a) Do you suffer from food cravings or bingeing?

▶ NO ▶ ▶ ▶

▼

YES

▼

b) Are you trying to diet to lose weight?

▶ NO ▶ ▶ ▶

▼

YES

▼

c) Do your family and friends tell you that you are not overweight, but underweight instead?

▶ NO ▶ ▶ ▶

▼

YES

▼

You might be suffering from anorexia/bulimia. See your doctor. If you are you can combine orthodox treatment with complementary therapies. Rejoin the chart for further advice.

Anorexia and bulimia

These are potentially fatal illnesses and require professional treatment. You should see your doctor about your eating problem before consulting this chart:
• If your weight is under 41kg (91lb) (female) and 51kg (112lb) (male).

• If you control your weight either by vomiting, or by using diuretics or laxatives.
• If you have a low body weight or little appetite and are in the habit of exercising strenuously.

go to next page

4

Are your cravings triggered by missing or delaying a meal?

NO ▶

▼
YES
▼

The cravings may be being triggered by low blood sugar (hypoglycemia).
An anti-hypoglycemic diet can help at a physical level. Try a therapy that focuses on nutrition, e.g. Class 14. On an energy-healing level, therapies that can stabilize the etheric body, such as Class 2 and 8 are useful.

5

Does emotional stress and/or worry trigger your eating problem? Do you "comfort eat"?

NO ▶

▼
YES
▼

Overeating, craving, or bingeing is how some people dampen down stress effects. The emotional body is disturbed and this filters down to the physical. Eating has a quieting effect on the physical, which can temporarily dampen down the emotional.
To avoid this, consider a therapy that puts you in touch with your emotional body and its needs (Class 5, 6, or 11). The same therapies may help under-eating when stressed. In this case the activation of the emotional body suppresses the free energy flow in the etheric and physical bodies, manifesting as loss of appetite. The latter is a healthy response as long as the stress does not become chronic.

You may be dieting too rigorously or changing your diet too quickly. Your etheric, and probably also your emotional body, cannot cope with this rate of change. Review your dieting plan. Eat more at each meal and snack on fruit. *Therapies that support the etheric body during a dietary change are Classes 2, 8, and 14. Class 3 techniques, supporting all subtle bodies, can also be useful, as well as Class 4 disciplines. Psychological support from a Class 11 therapy is particularly good for helping disturbances to the emotional body that dieting activates.*

Medical causes of obesity

There are few illnesses that result in being overweight. The most common is hypothyroidism. If you suspect you have an illness as well as a weight problem, consult your doctor before following this chart. Some drugs can cause obesity, e.g. some antidepressants, lithium, steroids, and for some people, the contraceptive pill. This is in part because the drugs affect the metabolism, but also they tend to increase appetite, either directly or because you feel better in yourself. If you suspect that a drug you are taking is making you put on weight consult your doctor. It may be possible to alter your treatment, but your only option may be to check your appetite and eat a lighter diet to combat the problem.

EATING DISORDERS/2

6

Does your eating problem (usually craving or bingeing) involve any or all of the following: chocolate, breads, cakes/biscuits, dairy foods, sweets? ▸ **NO** ▸

▼
YES
▼

This is typical of a food sensitivity. It can be a disturbance of any of the subtle bodies, but ultimately affecting the etheric and physical bodies.
See Food sensitivities chart, p. 180.

7

Are you "psychic" or over-sensitive to other people's emotions? ▸ **NO** ▸

▼
YES
▼

This can cause a difficulty with weight. It is the body's way of protecting the emotional body from subtle external energy fields. Treatments or disciplines that help stabilize your emotional body will make physical (weight) protection less necessary and you will find it becomes easier to lose weight.
Consider a Class 3, 4, 11, or 12 technique.

8

Have you seriously analyzed how much you eat? That is, have you kept a food diary for a week and recorded everything that enters your mouth, and the amounts? ▸ **NO** ▼

▼
YES
▼

Go to question 9 (below).

◂ ◂ ◂ ◂ ◂ ◂ ◂ ◂ ◂ ◂ ▼

▼

Keep a food diary for a week. Let a health professional advise you whether your food intake is in excess of your needs for your height/age/activity.

9

Are you eating less than expected for your height/age/weight? ▸ **NO** ▸

▼
YES
▼

Assuming you do not have an illness, such as thyroidism, and are not taking drugs that affect weight, you may be suffering from a food sensitivity (see p.180). This is especially likely if you feel bloated. Abstaining from the offending food(s) may dramatically improve your weight loss.

You have developed eating habits that oversupply your needs. To lose weight effectively and maintain weight loss your attitude to eating must change. *Class 11 techniques can help you achieve this. Also consider Class 14 therapies, as these can suggest a diet specific to your needs, together with treatments to help you align your subtle bodies. This will help you feel more comfortable in your being and more able to adjust to a new regime. The disciplines of Class 4 can help you maintain this.*

INDIGESTION/1

Indigestion is a symptom that can have many causes, ranging from a simple dietary indiscretion, through hiatus hernia, or peptic ulcers, to stomach cancer. Indigestion in under-40 year-olds is rarely cancer.

However, any persistent or recurrent digestive symptom that is not helped by dietary change or over-the-counter medicine should be discussed with your doctor.

1 Have you recently started a new medication? ▸ **NO** ▸

▼
YES
▼

Many medicines, particularly NSAIDs (anti-inflammatory painkillers) and aspirin can cause indigestion. See your doctor. You may need to change your medication or the times at which you are taking it. Medication affects the body at a physical level.
Rejoin this chart if this does not help.

2 Are you pregnant?

▼
YES
▼

The hormonal changes of pregnancy may cause indigestion. Pressure on the digestive system caused by the enlarging uterus later in pregnancy also aggravates the condition.
As this is a natural process you should try supportive treatment, good eating habits, or the Hay diet (see p.176).
If these do not help try a Class 2, 8, or 14 therapy to work with the etheric body and lessen its response to the hormonal changes.

▸ **NO** ▸ **3** Do you regularly succumb to one or more of the following bad eating habits: ▸ **NO** ▸

- Snack eating?
- Eating while standing up?
- Eating while working or at your desk?
- Eating less than 2 hours before going to bed?
- Eating little all day and then a large evening meal?
- Over-eating?
- Bolting your food?

▼
YES
▼

There are many entirely physical causes for indigestion. Good eating patterns will avoid these. As this is an abuse of the physical body it is inappropriate to use a healing method to override this.
However a Class 11 technique to help you to change your attitudes to eating may help. This works at the level of the mental body. If you still have this problem after adjusting your eating habits, rejoin the chart.

go to next page

ORTHODOX TREATMENTS

The treatment of indigestion has changed radically since the introduction of drugs that prevent the acid secretion in the stomach. In itself this acid is not necessarily the cause of indigestion as it has been discovered that a bacterium, *H. pylori*, is responsible for many cases.
As well as these treatments, old-fashioned antacids are often used for indigestion. They are safe and cheap, but do need to be taken regularly to be effective. As always, the side effects of these drugs,

such as diarrhoea, can be a problem and the long-term effects of the acid-blocking drugs is not yet known.
Many people with digestive problems feel that indigestion relates to their diet and the addition of something more to the diet may not be the best way to alleviate it. Often indigestion is obviously related to stress. Lack of stress and a good diet are important aspects of energy healing. Hence many people look to energy healing to help in this area.

INDIGESTION/2

4 ▶ NO ▶

Are you over 50 years old, and have you gradually noticed that you don't seem to digest food as well as you used to?

▼

YES

▼

With age, the digestive system becomes physically less efficient. *Energy-healing methods, especially Class 2, 8, and 14 therapies, working at the level of the etheric body, should help. Physically supportive treatments, such as digestive supplements and the Hay diet (see box, p.176), are very useful. They can help improve overall wellbeing as well as digestion, even though their primary effect is at the physical level.*

5 ▶ NO ▶

Are you overweight?

▼

YES

▼

The physical effects of being overweight tend to push the stomach up into the chest, creating a hiatus hernia. First try to lose weight; if you cannot, despite good eating habits, maybe your food preferences are not suiting you.
Try a Class 14 therapy. This may help you to pick up hidden food sensitivities (see chart, p.180). The Hay diet can also help (see box, p.176). These approaches work at a physical level and may help with weight loss as well as improving digestive problems.

6 ▶ NO ▶ ▶ ▶

Is your spine tender at the same level as the pain?

▼

YES

▼

Your indigestion may be due to irritation of the nerves that supply the stomach as they leave the spinal cord. This is due to a light vertebral displacement that impinges upon the nerves.
This can often be helped on a physical level by a Class 1 manipulation therapy.

7

▶ ▶ ▶ Do you find that certain foods do not "suit" you?

▼
YES
▼

This can be an indication of food sensitivities, often not to the foods that seem to disagree. It is more likely to be to foods consumed regularly, such as bread, wheat, or dairy foods. *Consider an elimination diet to identify suspects under the guidance of a Class 14 therapist with an interest in food intolerance. Removal of foods to which you are sensitive relieves stress on the digestive system and difficult-to-digest foods are tolerated. The Hay diet can also help relieve stress on the digestive system (see box, p.176). These changes act primarily at a physical level. Class 2 and 8 therapies may also help by stimulating the etheric body to work more efficiently. This filters through to the physical body. Class 14 therapies that focus on diet are also helpful.*

8

▶ NO ▶ Do you find that your symptoms are related to feeling stressed, either mentally, physically, or emotionally?

▼
YES
▼

The fear that stress generates in the emotional body directs the energy of the body away from the physical processes of digestion. This lowers the efficiency of the digestive process. To support yourself under stress, have a warm drink or soup and wait for your appetite to return before eating. If this problem is recurrent you might try a psychological approach.
Choose a Class 11 therapy to help you relax and to work with your belief systems (mental body) and your emotions (emotional body). Other therapies that may help are Class 3 therapies that affect the whole of the subtle body system and Class 2 and 8 therapies, which primarily affect the etheric body but influence the mental and emotional bodies. See also Anxiety chart (p.130).

9

▶ NO ▶ Do you find it difficult to express your true feelings or to accept criticism?

▼
YES
▼

This causes stress in the emotional body that filters down to affect the etheric and physical bodies.
Psychological techniques, such as Class 11 therapies, are useful to affect the emotional body. Methods that aim to release emotional energy trapped in the physical body might be even better. Consider Class 5, 6, or 7 therapies.

▶ NO ▶

go to next page

INDIGESTION/3

⑩

Are you anxious or depressed?

▼

YES

▼

These conditions, generated in the mental and emotional bodies, strongly affect the etheric body and via this, the physical body. The psychological state is where help is primarily needed.

To help the belief systems of the mental and emotional bodies, consider a Class 11 psychological therapy. Otherwise try a Class 2, 8, or 14 therapy to affect the etheric body primarily and, via this, the mental and emotional bodies. Class 3 therapies, affecting all the subtle bodies, are also useful as they help bring the whole being back into alignment with the causal body.

⑪

▶ NO ▶ **Is there a person or situation that you have difficulty in relating to, or that you feel insecure with, or anxiety about?**

▼

YES

▼

This stresses the energy centre at the solar plexus level. The disturbance is primarily at the etheric level, but filters to the physical level as indigestion. It may pass to the emotional level, generating fear or anger. You need to protect yourself better from the energy of the person or situation.

Class 11 therapies can do this. Class 3 healing methods are good, affecting all the subtle bodies and re-establishing your link with the causal body. A Class 13 power object may also help.

▶ NO ▶ *If you have come to the end of this chart without finding a possible cause, consult your doctor again. If no physical cause can be found, try a Class 2, 8, or 14 therapy. Your etheric body may be still experiencing the effects of a past trauma and these classes of therapy work on the etheric body to release this continuing need for symptoms.*

If this does not help, you may need to look into yourself more deeply, as the indigestion may be an indication that you need to change your belief system and mental body. This may be preventing a deep change in consciousness from happening. Such changes have the potential to affect all your subtle bodies as well as the physical body. The therapies most likely to help you in this process are Class 3, 7, 11, and 12, as they aim to connect you more closely with your causal body.

The Hay diet/food-combining

Food-combining began with the Hay diet, developed by Dr Hay in the 1920s. He considered this regime easy for the digestive system to handle and for the body to assimilate. Its basic principles are:

1. Cut down on "acid"-forming foods (proteins and starches).
2. Eliminate highly processed foods, as these are excessively acid-forming and poor sources of vitamins and minerals.
3. "Alkali"-forming foods (vegetables, salad, fruit) should form the bulk of the diet.

4. Eat starches at separate meals from proteins, as these foods are digested in different ways and mixing them leads to indigestion.

• Some Hay practitioners also consider that fruits should only be eaten between meals.
• The diet does not readily adapt to a vegetarian diet as pulses and soya products are not considered to be digestible foods.
• The diet is particularly useful for those with weight or digestive problems, or those who feel generally low in energy.

BOWEL DISORDERS/1

IRRITABLE BOWEL SYNDROME, CONSTIPATION, DIARRHOEA, WIND, BLOATING,
URGENCY TO DEFAECATE, ULCERATIVE COLITIS, AND CROHN'S DISEASE

Irritable bowel syndrome, with its many variations, is a disturbance of the digestive tract, with no serious long-term effects. However, ulcerative colitis and Crohn's disease are serious problems and can greatly undermine health. You will need carefully to combine orthodox with energy therapies, at least initially.

❶

Is your major problem constipation or an unsatisfactory bowel movement?

▼
YES
▼

This is likely to be due mainly to a problem at the physical level, so physical adjustments such as increasing your water and fibre intake, especially fruit and vegetables, and increasing exercise will all help. Note also any medication you are taking, as constipation is a side effect of many drugs (e.g. painkillers and iron supplements). On an energetic level the etheric body is disturbed.
This can be best helped by a Class 2, 8, or 14 therapy. Class 4 therapies would also be beneficial, especially yoga and tai chi, as on a physical level they stimulate the abdominal organs as well as having an effect on the subtle bodies.

❷

▸ NO ▸ Did your bowel problem follow a bout of gastro-enteritis, gastric 'flu, or a course of antibiotics?

▼
YES
▼

This problem is likely to be at the physical level, primarily due to a disturbance to the natural bacteria colonies found in the large bowel (see Bowel dysbiosis box, p. 178). The presence of abnormal bacteria or yeast disturbs the bowel at the etheric level as well.
This can be helped by homeopathy (Class 8) and Class 2 therapies. Class 3 and 14 therapies can also be useful, re-aligning the subtle bodies, which can be upset by an acute illness.

❸

▸ NO ▸ Does your bowel problem become worse when you are in stressful situations that upset you emotionally?

▼
YES
▼

The over-reaction of your emotional and probably also your mental body (stress challenges belief systems held in the mental body) is filtering down to disturb the etheric and physical bodies. *Consider a Class 2, 8, or 14 therapy. Although these work primarily at the etheric level they should be sufficiently penetrative of the emotional body to help the overall situation considerably. If the problem is deep-seated in the mental or emotional body a therapy focusing on those bodies may be more effective. Try a Class 11 technique. This should help you manage stress better, which is also a benefit from Class 4 and 6 therapies. Finally, Class 3 therapies allow the re-aligning of all subtle bodies – a common disturbance that stress produces.*

▸ NO ▸

go to next page

BOWEL DISORDERS/2

4 Did your bowel problem follow or occur during a period of stress or major life changes? ▶ NO ▶

5 If you are a woman, do your bowel problems relate to menstruation? ▶ NO ▶

6  Do you have back problems or other symptoms, such as headaches or sciatica, that relate to the working of the spine? ▶ NO ▶ ▶ ▶

YES
▼

This has caused an over-reaction in your emotional body – probably as a result of conflicts with beliefs held in the mental body. This emotional response has not been processed in a conscious way and has instead filtered down to affect the etheric and physical bodies.
Therapies that concentrate on the emotional body will be particularly beneficial as they will reveal to you what your underlying feelings are and allow you to deal with them in a conscious and healthier way.
Consider Class 5, 6, 7, or 11 therapies, as all your subtle bodies may have been disturbed by the stress. A Class 3 or 12 technique, which helps all the subtle bodies re-align, is useful.

YES
▼

The uterus is close to the bowel and can irritate it during menstruation – particularly causing diarrhoea. Also the hormonal changes of the cycle affect overall muscle tone and this affects the bowel's function. Your bowel disturbance is secondary to the physical and etheric changes in your body that relate to the hormone changes.
See the PMS chart (p. 159) as your bowel problems are part of this complex of symptoms.

YES
▼

You may have a chronic displacement of one or more facets of your vertebrae, which can disturb nerve supply to the digestive system. This is common and disturbs the working of the connection between the small and large bowel.
Try a Class 1 technique. This is a physical and etheric body disturbance.

Bowel dysbiosis

Once a bowel disorder has become established the natural bowel bacteria become disturbed, as they are unable to tolerate the abnormal bowel conditions. They are replaced by unhealthy organisms that like the disturbed bowel habit. These appear to secrete chemicals that encourage the bowel to perpetuate this state. For a treatment to have a long-term effect on the bowel the normal bowel "flora" need to become re-established, as these secrete chemicals that encourage normal bowel function. It can be very useful to supplement whatever energy treatment you have chosen with appropriate supplementation that helps achieve this. There is a wide number of options, for example acidophilus or lactobacillus preparations, linseed, grapefruit seed extract, pau d'arco tea or aloe vera juice, as well as herbal preparations. Supplements should be continued for at least 6 weeks.

(7)

▶ Do your symptoms come on unpredictably? Do you find yourself avoiding certain foods to try to control your symptoms?

▼
YES
▼

This is probably an etheric body disturbance and may be manifesting physically as food intolerance, but not necessarily to the foods you suspect (see Food sensitivities chart, p. 180). However, beware of over-restricting your diet as this can become a problem in itself. *Therapies such as Class 2 or 8 therapies, which tackle this problem at the etheric level, can relieve the need to avoid foods. Other therapies that work at more levels can also be beneficial, especially Classes 3 and 11, as food intolerance is usually complex and involves disturbances at all levels. These types of allergic problem, particularly if extensive, may also benefit from a Class 9 approach. Allergy-based symptoms often need more physical support than just food avoidance. Class 14 remedies are useful in this way.*

▶ NO ▶ *If you have come to the end of this chart without identifying a cause try a Class 2, 8, or 14 therapy, which focus on the etheric body. If this does not help then look inside yourself more deeply to find out more about what your bowel problem may represent, particularly with reference to your belief systems and mental body. You may be having difficulty making changes in your beliefs, preventing deep changes in consciousness from happening. Such changes could help all your subtle bodies as well as the physical body. The therapies most likely to help are Class 3, 11, and 12 therapies.*

WARNING

Bowel problems, especially occurring for the first time in the over-35s, that show blood in the stool, are persistent, or make you feel generally unwell, should be discussed with your doctor before you consider alternative treatments. If you develop any of the following symptoms, see your doctor:

● You are over 40 and you develop a new bowel symptom.
● You develop constant abdominal pain, diarrhoea, or abdominal distention.
● You pass blood in your stool.
● You are losing weight.

ORTHODOX TREATMENTS

Irritable bowel syndrome is notoriously difficult to treat with orthodox medicine. Dietary changes, such as increasing fibre, changing to non-wheat fibre, avoiding dairy products or excess caffeine or alcohol, are often suggested in preference to drugs. The most common medications are bulking agents. The main drugs are anti-spasmodics, which relax the gut wall. Ulcerative colitis and Crohn's disease are rarer and more serious, needing orthodox diagnosis. When active they need orthodox treatment as they can be life-threatening, though they are chronic diseases, which go through good and bad periods. The main drugs are steroids, aminosalicylates, immuno-suppressives, antidiarrhoeals, and sometimes antibiotics. Surgery is sometimes needed. Many of the drugs can cause side effects. Diverticular disease is treated the same as irritable bowel syndrome, but can develop complications, needing hospital treatment. Coeliac disease is treated solely by dietary means – a gluten-free diet. Coeliac is a life-long condition. With age, there is a risk of small bowel cancers and lymphomas if the diet has not been followed.

FOOD SENSITIVITIES/1

1

Do you get a vigorous (anaphylactic) reaction to a food shortly after eating it? This might include nettle rash, swelling, or wheezing. Even very small amounts of the food may precipitate a reaction.

▼
YES
▼

This is a true allergy to food, known as an anaphylactic reaction. It can be life-threatening and you should see your doctor about it. You may need to carry emergency adrenaline in case you have an attack. This reaction may be modified by using classes of treatments that work well on the etheric body, where this reaction originates.
Consider a Class 2, 8, or 14 therapy.

▶ NO ▶

2

a) Did your symptoms dramatically improve when you removed a suspected food from your diet?

▼
YES
▼

b) Have you tried re-introducing the food, or foods?

▼
YES
▼
▼

c) Are you "allergic" only to dairy foods? And are your symptoms related to digestion?

▼
YES
▼

You may have an intolerance to milk sugar (lactose).
Try using lactose supplements and keeping dairy to a minimum. Many adults lose their childhood tolerance to lactose as the enzyme that breaks it down is no longer present in adulthood. This is especially common in non-caucasians. If this does not help, rejoin the chart.

▶ NO ▶

▶ NO ▶

You should make sure your symptoms are related to foods before continuing with this chart. *See Elimination diet box, p.182.*

▼
YES
▼

You should do so, otherwise the improvements may be coincidental and nothing to do with the food (see Elimination diet box, p. 182). *Once you have done this, return to the chart.*

3

Did your intolerance to foods seem to appear after any of the following:
● Treatment with oral steroids?
● Treatment with frequent or long-term antibiotics?
● Childbirth?
● Gastroenteritis or gastric 'flu?

▼
YES
▼

These can all upset the natural bacterial population of your lower bowel (see Bowel dysbiosis box, p. 178), making the wall more permeable to foods and triggering sensitivities.
Food supplements and herbs (Class 14) can help. Other classes that are useful are those that affect the etheric body, for example Classes 2 and 8. If you also have a back problem, Class 1 manipulation therapies may help.

▶ NO ▶ ▶ ▶

4

▶ Did your problems begin after moving house – especially if other members of your household also suffered from ill health or psychological difficulties?

▼
YES
▼

Your house may be affected by geopathic stress. These disturbances in the subtle energies of your environment may be affecting your own etheric body, which is precipitating food sensitivity reactions.
Try a Class 9 technique.

▶ **NO** ▶

5

Have you been vegetarian for some time?

▼
YES
▼

The staples of vegetarian diets – grains and dairy foods – are very prone to triggering food sensitivities. Also the restriction of foods available, if these foods as well as animal products are removed from the diet, can amplify the problem, as you may become more and more sensitive to the foods you are eating.
A therapy that acts on the etheric body, such as a Class 2, 8, 11, or 14 therapy, would be a useful approach.

▶ **NO** ▶

6

Are you generally very sensitive to your environment and the presence of others. Does this cause emotional strains?

▼
YES
▼

This sensitivity may be spreading to your foods. It is important that you strengthen the boundaries of your energy field, particularly at the emotional level.
Class 11 psychotherapies and Class 3 healing methods can be useful.
You may also need support for your etheric body.
Class 2, 8, and 14 therapies are useful both at the etheric and emotional level. Class 13 techniques can also help with this protection.

▶ **NO** ▶

go to next page

FOOD SENSITIVITIES/2

7

Have you been exposed to large, or constant small levels, of environmental toxins such as organophosphate pesticides or chemicals at work.

▶ NO ▶

▼
YES
▼

These chemicals damage the immune system and so trigger food and environmental sensitivity. This particularly affects the etheric and physical bodies. Therapies that strengthen the immune system may be helpful.
Consider Class 2, 8, and 14 therapies.

8

Do you find it difficult to cope with changes in your routine or lifestyle?

▶ NO ▶

▼
YES
▼

Fear, often coupled with a need to be in control, may be affecting you, not just emotionally but also physically, producing food sensitivities. The sensitivities are affecting both your emotional and etheric bodies, possibly also the mental body.
Consider Class 3 methods to connect you to your causal body and so lessen fear. Also consider Class 11 psychological techniques. If you have difficulty expressing emotions physically Class 5 and 6 therapies may be useful.

If you cannot find a reason why you might be suffering from food allergies, see your doctor to make sure that there is no other physical cause. Many orthodox practitioners are sceptical about the existence of food allergies, so it is important to verify that a food or foods are causing the problem. At the other extreme there are some practitioners of complementary medicine who consider that a very large proportion of symptoms are due to food or chemical sensitivities. Be careful not to exclude too many foods without professional supervision. If you do have food sensitivities there will be an underlying cause, likely to be connected to an inner need for changes in consciousness arising from your connection with your causal body. To do this you may need to change your belief systems, which relate to your mental body. Changes here can filter through the rest of the subtle bodies to the physical and so relieve the food allergies. Therapies that are most able to help include Classes 3, 7, 11, and 12.

Elimination diet

To check if a food is causing you a problem eliminate it entirely from your diet for 2 to 4 weeks. At the end of this time reintroduce the food in normal quantities back into your diet. Note if any of your symptoms return. Do this for a week before deciding if the food is not suiting you. You need to exclude ALL products that contain the food you are testing. The commonest foods to cause sensitivities are dairy products, wheat, yeasts, sugars, and caffeine, but any commonly eaten food may be a problem.

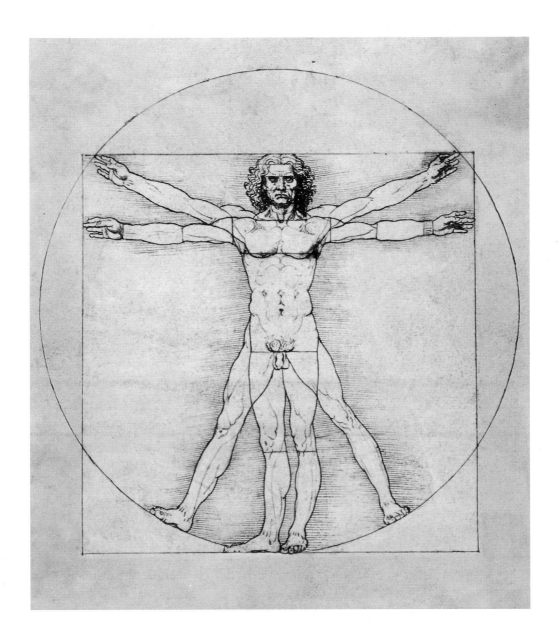

RESOURCES

Anthroposophy
Anthroposophical Therapy
and Hygiene Association
(ANTHA)
241 Hungry Hollow Road
Spring Valley, NY 10977

Anthroposophical Society in
America
1923 Gedes Avenue
Ann Arbor, MI 48104-1797
(734) 662-9355
information@anthroposophy.com

Physicians Association for
Anthroposophical Medicine
PO Box 269
Kimberton, PA 19442

Applied kinesiology
International College of
Applied Kinesiology
ICAKUSA Central Office
6405 Metcalf Avenue
Suite 503
Shawnee Mission, KS 66202
(913) 384-5336

Touch For Health
Kinesiology Association
11262 Washington Blvd.
Culver City, CA 90230
(800) 466-8342

Autogenic training
Ruth Benor
Medford, MA 02155
(609) 714-1885

Bach flower remedies
Nelson Bach USA, Ltd.
Wilmington Technology Park
100 Research Drive
Wilmington, MA 01887-4406
(800) 334-0843

Flower Essence Society
PO Box 1769
Nevada City, CA 95959
(916) 265-0258
mail@flowersociety.org
www.flowersociety.org

Biodynamic massage
American Alliance of
Massage Professionals
3108 Rte 10 West
Denville, NJ 07834

American Institute of
Massage Therapy
2156 Newport Boulevard
Costa Mesa, CA 92627

American Massage Therapy
Association
820 Davis Street
Suite 100
Evanston, IL 60201

Healing Hands Institute for
Massage Therapy
41 Bergline Avenue
Westwood, NJ 07675

Chi kung
Qigong Institute/East West
Academy of the Healing Arts
450 Sutter Street
Suite 916
San Francisco, CA 94108

Qigong Universal
2828 Beverly Boulevard
Los Angeles, CA 90057

National Qigong (Chi Kung)
Association
PO Box 20218
Boulder Springs, CO 80308
(888) 218-7788
info@nqa.org

Chinese herbalism
American Foundation of
Traditional Chinese Medicine
505 Beach Street
San Francisco, CA 94133
(415) 776-0502

Color therapy
Harmony Institute of Light
PO Box 924
Kihei, HI 96753
(808) 879-3737
harmony@maui.com

Crystal Healing
The Crystal Academy of
Advanced Healing Arts
PO Box 1334
Kapaa, HI 96746
(808) 823-6959

Bioenergy Fields Foundation
PO Box 4234
Malibu, CA 90265
(310) 457-4694

Dowsing
American Society of
Dowsers
PO Box 24
Danville, VT 05828
(800) 711-9530

Eurythmy
Eurythmy Spring Valley
260 Hungry Hollow Road
Chestnut Ridge, NY 10977
(914) 352-5020 ext 13
eury@mail.creativeonline.com

Feldenkrais method
The Feldenkrais Guild
PO Box 489
Albany, OR 97321-0143
(800) 775-2118

Feldenkrais Resources
830 Bancroft Way #112
Berkeley, CA 94710
(800) 765-1907

Feng shui
Feng Shui Warehouse
PO Box 3005
San Diego, CA 92163

Feng Shui Institute of
America
PO Box 488
Wabasso, FL 32970

Five rhythms dance™
The Moving Center School
Mill Valley, CA 94941
(413) 388-0431
info@movingcenterschool.com

Hypnotherapy
Academy for Guided Imagery
PO Box 2070
Mill Valley, CA 94942

American Association of
Professional
Hypnotherapists
PO Box 29
Boones Mill, VA 24065

American Society for
Clinical Hypnosis
2200 East Devon Avenue
Suite 291
Des Plaines, IL 600118

National Guild of Hypnotists
PO Box 308
Merrimack, NH 03054

Meditation
Insight Meditation Society
1230 Pleasant Street
Barre, MA 01005
(617) 355-4378

Spirit Rock
5000 Sir Francis Drake
Boulevard
PO Box 909
Woodacre, CA 94973
(415) 488-0164

Zen Centre of San Francisco
300 Page Street
San Francisco, CA 94102
(415) 863-3136

Neurolinguistic programming
The NLP Center of New York
24 E 12th Street
Suite 402
New York, NY 10003
(212) 647-0860
NLP@Earthlink.net
www.nlptraining.com

NLP Information Center
www.nlpinfo.com
info@nlpinfo.com

Psychoanalysis
American Academy of
Psychoanalysis
47 East 19th Street
6th Floor
New York, NY 10003-1323
(212) 475-7980
aapnatoff@aol.com
http://aapsa.org

The American
Psychoanalytic Association
309 East 49th Street
New York, NY 10017
(212) 752-0450
central.office@apsa.org
www.apsa.org

Re-evaluation counselling
American Counseling
Association
5999 Stevenson Avenue
Alexandria, VA 22304-3300

Reiki
www.reikilinks.com

Rolfing®
The Rolf Institute
205 Canyon Boulevard
Boulder, CO 80302
(303) 449-5903
rolf.institute@rolf.org
www.rolf.org

Shamanic healing
Dancing Bear Alternative
Health Center
1000 Fremont Avenue
Suite 150c
Los Altos, CA 95134
(650) 947-8980
www.dancing-bear.com

Shiatsu
Boston Shiatsu School
1972 Massachusetts Avenue
Cambridge, MA 02140
(617) 876-4048
www.bostonshiatsu.nv.
switchboard.com

Sound therapy
Casa de Maria Research
Center
8811 53rd Avenue W.
Mukilteo, WA 98275
(888) 262-8348
www.napanet.net/~mmst/

Kairos Institute of Sound
Healing, LLC
(206) 720 6198
www.kairos-institute.com

American Music Therapy
Association Inc.
8455 Colesville Road
Suite 1000
Silver Spring, MD 20910
(301) 589-3300
info@musictherapy.org
www.musictherapy.org

Spiritual healing
Spiritual Healing Common
Boundary, Inc.
7005 Florida Street
Chevy Chase, MD 20815

Order of the Ascending Spirit
9120 Gramercy Drive #317
San Diego, CA 92123-4010
(615) 560-9228
http:dharma-haven.org/oas

Tai chi
Tai Chi Center of New York
125 West 43rd Street
New York, NY 10036
(212) 221-6110
www.chutaichi.com

Trance dance
The Moving Center
PO Box 271
New York, NY 10276
(973) 642-1979

Zero balancing
The Zero Balancing
Association
PO Box 1727
Capitola, CA 95010
(831) 476-0665
info@zerobalancing.com
www.zerobalancing.com

BIBLIOGRAPHY

Brennan, Barbara Ann, *Hands of Light: A Guide to Healing Through the Human Energy Field*, Bantam Books, 1987

Chevallier, Andrew, *Encyclopedia of Medicinal Plants*, Dorling Kindersley, 1996

Cummings, David, *Handbook for Light Workers*, Barton House, 1993

Dewhurst-Maddock, *Healing with Sound*, Simon and Schuster, 1993

Douglas-Klotz, *Prayers of the Cosmos*, Harper, 1994

Evans, Dr Michael, and Rodger, Iaian, *Anthroposophical Medicine – Treating Body, Soul and Spirit*, Floris Books, 1998

Feldenkrais, Moshe, *Awareness Through Movement*, Penguin, 1990

Feldenkrais, Moshe, *The Elusive Obvious*, Meta, 1989

Gardner, Kay, *Sounding the Inner Landscape – Music as Medicine*, Element, 1997

Gibran, Kahlil, *The Prophet*, Penguin, 1998

Goldman, Jonathan, *Healing Sounds: The Power of Harmonics*, Element, 1996

Hoffman, David, *The Herbal Handbook*, Healing Arts Press, 1998

Iyengar, B.S.K., *Light on Pranayama*, Aquarian, 1992

Johari, Harish, *The Healing Power of Gemstones*, Healing Arts Press, 1996

Kam Chuen, Master Lam, *The Way of Energy*, Simon and Schuster, 1991

Mercarti, Maria, *The Handbook of Chinese Massage*, Healing Arts Press, 1997

Ray, Sondra, *Celebration of Breath*, Celestial Arts, 1984

Réquéna, Yves, *Chi Kung*, Healing Arts Press, 1997

Roth, Gabrielle, *Maps to Ecstasy*, Thorsons, 1999

Rowland, Amy, *Traditional Reiki for Our Times*, Healing Arts Press, 1998

Rutherford, Leo, *Principles of Shamanism*, Thorsons, 1997

Scheffer, Mechthild, *Bach Flower Therapy*, Healing Arts Press, 1988

Simpson, Liz, *The Book of Crystal Healing*, Gaia Books, 1997

Steiner, Rudolf, *How to Know the Higher Worlds*, Anthroposophic Press, 1994

Steiner, Rudolf, *Knowledge of the Higher Worlds*, Anthroposophic Press, 1994

Thie, John, *Touch for Health*, Devorss, 1973

Valentine, Tom and Carol, *Applied Kinesiology*, Healing Arts Press, 1987

Wood, Betty, *The Healing Power of Color*, Healing Arts Press, 1998

GLOSSARY

Astral body
The emotional body.

Aura
Energy field surrounding the body. Includes all areas of the field, but the innermost etheric and emotional bodies are the easiest to discern.

Causal body
Outermost part of the energy field, connecting with the universal energy field, or "divine" or Higher Self – source of intuition/inspiration.

Chakra
Sanskrit for "wheel". Seen as spinning light, linking the subtle bodies and connecting them to the physical body. Considered energy centres, or vortices of energy, within the subtle bodies.

Chi
Chinese term for the universal energy underlying the physical Universe. Our bodies are made up of chi, animated by it, needing a free flow of chi for good health.

Emotional body
Area of the body's energy field lying between the etheric and mental bodies. Related to our emotional state – the part of ourselves thought to be capable of separating from the physical body, as in dreaming or out-of-body experiences.

Etheric body
Innermost part of the body's energy field. Closely linked to the physical body, disturbances in this correspond to problems in the physical body. Can be likened to a blueprint of the physical body that forms a force field within which the physical body condenses.

Health body
The etheric body.

Higher Self
The causal body.

Kundalini
Subtle energy considered to lie at the root chakra. It can rise through the chakras, ultimately reaching the crown. At each chakra there is transformation. At the crown there is enlightenment. Although liberating, its effects can be traumatic.

Life force
That which animates living organisms. Aspects of chi (Chinese), qi or Ki (Japanese), and prana (Sanskrit) are its Oriental equivalents. See also Universal life force.

Mental body
The area of the energy field surrounding the body that lies above the emotional and below the causal body. It is the area influenced by our thoughts and beliefs.

Meridians
Pathways of energy flow travelling along the body surface and through internal organs. The energy framework upon which Oriental medicine and related techniques are based.

Orthodox medicine
Modern medical practice based on drugs and surgery.

Prana
Sanskrit for "life breath". The life force that permeates all things. Equivalent to chi.

Sanskrit
An ancient language, the foundation of many modern languages. Hindu sacred texts are written in Sanskrit. The earliest of these, the Vedas, are over 4000 years old.

Subtle bodies
The layered energy field permeating and enveloping the physical body. It is thought to be made up of increasingly refined frequencies, which lie beyond what is measurable. The different bands of frequencies form the subtle bodies, each with different properties, and all essential for the development and maintenance of a complete human being.

Universal life force
The basic energy composing the whole manifest Universe, lying behind everything we are aware of. It is equivalent to the chi and prana of Eastern philosophies. When it animates a living organism it becomes life force.

The Vedas
Ancient spiritual texts, in Sanskrit, containing fundamental teaching from which Hinduism, ayurveda, and yoga developed. Likely also to be the source from which Taoism and traditional Oriental medicine developed. The roots of Western religions and philosophical thought may also have been influenced by them.

Yin and yang
Negative and positive polarizations of life energy, chi, which composes the manifest Universe. Everything contains yin and yang in varying proportions. The process of life constantly shifts the balance between them.

INDEX

Author's acknowledgments

I would like to acknowledge the following practitioners for the time and expertise that they gave so freely in order that I could portray their techniques in an authentic way. Many were friends before I started and others have become friends since. I hope that I have done their work justice.

Sonia Allen-Wall (yoga, pranayama, reflexology); Dr Graham Barrowcliffe (hypnotherapy); Jill Bird (autogenic training); Danny Blythe (tai chi); David Bolton (chi kung); Smadar Bronzi (eurythmy); Enid Bufton (spiritual healing); John Bullock (feng shui); James D'Angelo (sound therapy); Ann Casement (Jungian psychoanalysis); Andrew Chevallier (herbalism); Paul Cohen (zero balancing); Theolyn Cortens (prayer); Carol Crowell (therapeutic touch); Dr Jyoti Dattani (ayurveda); Dr Allyn Edwards (chiropractic); Dr Michael Evans (anthroposophy); Ron George (dowsing); Kardien Gerbrands (biodynamic massage); Theo Gimbel (colour therapy); David Glassman (Alexander technique, neurolinguistic programming); Jonathan Horowitz (shamanic healing); Avril Jacques (aromatherapy); Margot Messenger (rebirthing); Nicola Morgan (shiatsu); Terry Moule (naturopathy); Garet Newel (Feldenkrais method); Chris Robinson (applied kinesiology); Lynda Rolfe-Boulton (crystal healing); Alan Rudolf (Rolfing®); Leo Rutherford (five rhythms dance™, trance dance); Dr David Scott (meditation); Dale Spence (osteopathy); Ian Spiers (reiki); Keith Turner (re-evaluation counselling); Dr Philip Vernon (acupuncture, Chinese herbalism); Patrick Vickerman (dowsing).

Many of my friends, in one way or another, helped me to put this book together and I am grateful not only for their friendship but also for their constant interest and support. In particular I would like to thank Ann Casey, Joy Cole, Joanna Cross, Greg Fladager, Dr Peter Griffith, John Patmore, Jennie Powell, Martyn Rudin, and Sue Washington for their advice, loan of materials, and resources.

I have one person that needs very special acknowledgment – Cathy Meeus. It is through my friendship with her that this book came to be written. I would also like to thank my editors, Jo Godfrey Wood and Katherine Pate, for not only their editing but their encouragement and steadfastness during the process of producing this book.

Photographic credits

p 2 CERN/Science Photo Library (SPL); p 12 SPL/K. Kent; p 13 SPL/H. Dakin; pp 18–19 Delilah Dyson; p 23 SuperStock; p 24 Delilah Dyson; p 28 CERN/SPL/Patrice Loiez; p 34 SPL/Dr Yorgos Nikas; p 39 Telegraph Colour Library; p 42 Roland Sheridan/Ancient Art and Architecture; p 43 Durham University Library; p 44 Ancient Art and Architecture; p 47 Gaia Books; p 51 Delilah Dyson; p 55 Gaia Books/Steve Teague; pp 60–1 Gaia Books/Steve Teague; p 64 Delilah Dyson; p 68 Gaia Books/Fausto Dorelli; p 70 Gaia Books/Philip Dowell; p 76 Gaia Books/Fausto Dorelli; pp 80–1 Cliché Musées Nationaux/Documentation Photographique de la Réunion des Musées Nationaux; p 83 Gaia Books/Doug Baillie; pp 94–5 Gaia Books/Philip Dowell; p 96 Gaia Books/Fausto Dorelli; pp 101, 107 Delilah Dyson; p 116 Gaia Books/Fausto Dorelli; pp 118–54 Gaia Books/Steve Teague; p 155 Gaia Books/Justin Pumfrey; pp 156–82 Gaia Books/Steve Teague; p 183 SuperStock.

Publishers' acknowledgments

Gaia Books would like to thank the following for their help in the production of this book: Anne Brabyn (bibliography), Lynn Bresler (indexing and proofreading), Owen Dixon (design and production assistance), Max Drake, Delilah Dyson (photography), Mark Epton (design assistance), Tamsin Juggins (keying), Deborah Pate (keying), Mary Pickles (proofreading), Helena Petre (keying), Steve Teague (photography in Part Three), Colette Wilson (picture research).

For further reading

AMMA THERAPY
A Complete Textbook of Oriental Bodywork and Medical Principles
Tina Sohn and Robert Sohn
ISBN 0-89281-488-8 • $45.00 hardcover • 448 pages, 8¹/₂ x 11 • 170 b&w illustrations
This groundbreaking form of bodywork incorporates elements of acupuncture, herbalism, diet, and exercise to maintain the movement of life energy within the body.

TRADITIONAL REIKI FOR OUR TIMES
Practical Methods for Personal and Planetary Healing
Amy Z. Rowland
ISBN 0-89281-777-1 • $19.95 paperback • 256 pages, 8 x 10 • 80 b&w photographs
This comprehensive Reiki training manual progresses step-by-step through Reiki level I and II classes and shows how to set up a professional practice.

THE REFLEXOLOGY MANUAL
An Easy-to-Use Illustrated Guide to the Healing Zones of the Hands and Feet
Pauline Wills
ISBN 0-89281-547-7 • $19.95 paperback • 144 pages, 8¹/₂ x 11 • 150 color photographs

THE HANDBOOK OF CHINESE MASSAGE
Tui Na Techniques to Awaken Body and Mind
Maria Mercati
ISBN 0-89281-745-3 • $19.95 paperback • 7¹/₂ x 9⁵/₈ • 140 color photographs
An authority on Oriental massage integrates classic *tui na* techniques into a new, whole-body treatment never before seen in East or West.

THE BOOK OF KI
A Practical Guide to the Healing Principles of Life Energy
Mallory Fromm, Ph.D.
ISBN 0-89281-744-5 • $16.95 paperback • 128 pages, 7 x 10 • 68 b&w photographs
Simple exercises teach you to access and transmit your ki for optimum health.

CHINESE MASSAGE FOR INFANTS AND CHILDREN
Traditional Techniques for Alleviating Colic, Colds, Earaches, and Other Common Childhood Conditions
Kyle Cline
ISBN 0-89281-797-6 • $19.95 paperback • 160 pages, 8 x 10 • 180 b&w line drawings
A leading practitioner of Chinese medicine provides a handbook of simple massage techniques that parents can use to participate in their children's health care.

These and other Healing Arts Press/Inner Traditions titles are available at many fine bookstores, or, to order directly from the publisher, please send check or money order payable to Inner Traditions for the total amount, plus $3.50 shipping for the first book and $1.00 for each additional book to:

Inner Traditions, P.O. Box 388, Rochester, VT 05767
Fax (802) 767-3726 • Or call 1-800-246-8648
Visit our Web site: www.InnerTraditions.com